The Complete 30-Minute Renal Diet Cookbook

Delicious and Nutritious Kidney-Friendly Recipes Prepared in 30 Minutes or Less to Boost Your Wellness and Manage Kidney Diseases. Contains Low-Sodium, Low-Potassium, and Low-Phosphorus Recipes

Amanda K. Sanders

Amanda K. Sanders

© 2024 Amanda K. Sanders. All rights reserved.

No part of this book may be reproduced, distributed, or transmitted in any form or by any means, including photocopying, recording, or other electronic or mechanical methods, without the prior written permission of the publisher, except in the case of brief quotations embodied in critical reviews and certain other noncommercial uses permitted by copyright law.

Table of Contents

Introduction 1
    Understanding the Renal Diet 1

Chapter 1: Importance of Quick and Nutritious Meals and Efficient Cooking Tips 2
    Importance of Quick and Nutritious Meals 2
    Tips for Efficient Cooking 2

Chapter 2: 30-Day Meal Plan 4
    Meal Plan for Days 1-20 4
    Meal Plan for Days 21-30 5

Breakfast 7
    Yogurt and Berry Bowl 8
    Cinnamon Raisin French Toast 9
    Apple Cinnamon Oatmeal 10
    Blueberry Pancakes 11
    Banana Nut Muffins 12
    Greek Yogurt Parfait 13
    Vegetable Frittata 14
    Strawberry Banana Smoothie 15
    Avocado Toast 16
    Breakfast Quesadilla 17
    Spinach and Mushroom Omelette 18
    Whole Grain Waffles 19
    Breakfast Casserole 20

Lunch 21
    Turkey and Avocado Wrap 22
    Greek Salad 23
    Chicken Caesar Salad 24
    Quinoa Salad 25

Tuna Salad 26
Lentil Soup 27
Minestrone Soup 28
Black Bean Soup 29
Chicken Noodle Soup 30
Caprese Salad 31
Egg Salad Sandwich 32
Tomato Basil Soup 33
Greek Chickpea Salad 34
Vegetable Barley Soup 35
Chicken and Rice Soup 36
Spinach and Lentil Salad 37
Roasted Vegetable Wrap 38
Beef and Barley Soup 39

Dinner 40
Baked Salmon 41
Lemon Herb Chicken 42
Turkey Chili 43
Grilled Shrimp Skewers 44
Ratatouille 45
Chicken Stir-Fry 46
Beef Stew 47
Baked Cod 48
Pork Tenderloin 49
Vegetable Stir-Fry 50
Stuffed Peppers 51
Turkey Meatballs 52
Baked Chicken Parmesan 53
Lemon Garlic Tilapia 54
Beef and Broccoli 55

    Mushroom Risotto 56

    Spinach and Feta Stuffed Chicken 57

    Lentil Curry 58

Snacks 59

    Apple Slices with Peanut Butter 60

    Trail Mix 61

    Greek Yogurt 62

    Cheese and Crackers 63

    Rice Cakes with Hummus 64

    Mixed Nuts 65

    Carrot Sticks with Hummus 66

    Cottage Cheese 67

    Popcorn 68

    Sliced Cucumber with Lemon 69

    Fruit Salad 70

    Edamame 71

    Pretzels 72

    Roasted Chickpeas 73

    Yogurt Bark 74

    Peanut Butter Banana Bites 75

    Veggie Chips 76

Desserts 77

    Berry Crisp 78

    Poached Pears 79

    Rice Pudding 80

    Angel Food Cake 81

    Banana Ice Cream 82

    Strawberry Sorbet 83

    Chocolate Avocado Mousse 84

    Lemon Poppy Seed Muffins 85

Pumpkin Pie 86
  Oatmeal Raisin Cookies 87
  Peach Cobbler 88
  Apple Cinnamon Bars 89
  Coconut Macaroons 90
  Berry Smoothie Bowl 91
  Greek Yogurt Cheesecake 92
  Chocolate Covered Strawberries 93
  Chia Seed Pudding 94

Beverages 95
  Green Smoothie 96
  Iced Herbal Tea 97
  Fruit Infused Water 98
  Almond Milk 99
  Protein Shake 100
  Vegetable Juice 101
  Coconut Water 102
  Iced Coffee 103
  Golden Milk 104
  Sparkling Water 105
  Chai Latte 106
  Hot Chocolate 107
  Fresh Squeezed Juice 108
  Matcha Latte 109
  Kombucha 110
  Electrolyte Drink 111
  Horchata 112
  Soy Milk 113

Conclusion 114
  Tips for Maintaining a Renal-Friendly Diet 114

Meal Planning and Prep Ideas 114

Recipes Index.. 116

Introduction

Welcome to *"The Complete 30-Minute Renal Diet Cookbook"*! With this cookbook, you can prepare delicious and nutritious meals that support your kidney health in just 30 minutes or less. Cooking for a renal diet can be challenging, but with the right guidance and recipes, you can enjoy flavorful and satisfying meals without compromising your health. In this introduction, we'll explore the fundamentals of the renal diet, the importance of quick and nutritious meals, and tips for efficient cooking to make your time in the kitchen both enjoyable and productive.

Understanding the Renal Diet

The renal diet is specifically designed for individuals with chronic kidney disease (CKD) or those undergoing dialysis. This diet helps manage the balance of fluids, minerals, and electrolytes in your body, reducing the burden on your kidneys and preventing further damage. Key components of the renal diet include:

- **Low Sodium**: High sodium intake can increase blood pressure and cause fluid retention, which puts extra strain on your kidneys. Try to restrict your daily sodium intake to no more than 2,000 mg.

- **Controlled Protein**: While protein is essential for maintaining muscle mass and overall health, excessive protein can produce waste that your kidneys must filter. Balance your protein intake based on your chronic kidney disease (CKD) stage, and consult your healthcare provider for personalized recommendations.

- **Limited Potassium**: High potassium levels can cause heart problems and other complications. Monitor your intake of potassium-rich foods such as bananas, potatoes, and spinach.

- **Restricted Phosphorus**: Elevated phosphorus levels can lead to bone and heart issues. Limit dairy products, nuts, and processed foods that contain high amounts of phosphorus.

By adhering to these guidelines, you can help preserve kidney function and maintain overall health. This cookbook provides recipes that align with these dietary restrictions while offering variety and flavor.

This cookbook will inspire you to embrace the renal diet and discover the joy of cooking quick, nutritious meals. With some planning and the right recipes, you can make every meal a delightful and healthy experience. Let's begin this journey to better kidney health, one 30-minute meal at a time!

Chapter 1: Importance of Quick and Nutritious Meals and Efficient Cooking Tips

Importance of Quick and Nutritious Meals

In our fast-paced world, finding the time to prepare healthy meals can be challenging, especially when managing a chronic condition like CKD. Quick and nutritious meals are crucial for several reasons:

- **Time Management**: Cooking meals in 30 minutes or less allows you to balance your dietary needs with other responsibilities, whether you're working, caring for your family, or pursuing hobbies.

- **Consistent Nutrition**: Eating regular, balanced meals helps maintain energy levels, stabilize blood sugar, and support overall well-being. Quick meals reduce the temptation to opt for unhealthy convenience foods.

- **Stress Reduction**: Simplifying meal preparation can reduce stress and make cooking a more enjoyable experience. Knowing you can quickly prepare a healthy meal can provide peace of mind and improve your relationship with food.

- **Adherence to Dietary Restrictions**: A repertoire of quick, renal-friendly recipes can help you adhere to your dietary guidelines and avoid foods that could exacerbate your condition.

Tips for Efficient Cooking

To make the most of your time in the kitchen and ensure that your meals are both quick and nutritious, consider the following tips for efficient cooking:

1. **Plan Ahead**: Take time each week to plan your meals and create a shopping list. This will help you stay organized and ensure you have all the necessary ingredients on hand.

2. **Prep Ingredients in Advance**: Prepare vegetables, proteins, and other ingredients beforehand. Pre-chop vegetables, marinate proteins, and portion out spices to streamline the cooking process.

3. **Utilize Kitchen Tools**: Invest in time-saving kitchen tools such as a food processor, slow cooker, or pressure cooker. These appliances can significantly reduce prep and cooking time.

4. **Keep a Well-Stocked Pantry**: Stock up on renal-friendly staples such as low-sodium broths, canned vegetables (rinsed to reduce sodium), whole grains, and herbs and spices. Having these essentials on hand can make meal preparation faster and more convenient.

5. **Batch Cook**: Cook larger portions of meals and freeze leftovers for future use. This can save time on busy days and ensure you always have a healthy option available.

6. **Simplify Recipes**: Choose recipes with fewer ingredients and straightforward instructions. This will save time and reduce the likelihood of errors or complications while cooking.

7. **Stay Organized**: Keep your kitchen workspace clean and organized. A clutter-free environment makes finding what you need and working efficiently easier.

By following these tips, you'll be able to create delicious, renal-friendly meals in no time. This will support your health and allow you to enjoy the benefits of nutritious, home-cooked food.

Chapter 2: 30-Day Meal Plan

Meal Plan for Days 1-20

Day	Breakfast	Lunch	Dinner	Snacks
1	Yogurt and Berry Bowl	Turkey and Avocado Wrap	Baked Salmon	Apple Slices with Peanut Butter
2	Cinnamon Raisin French Toast	Greek Salad	Lemon Herb Chicken	Trail Mix
3	Apple Cinnamon Oatmeal	Chicken Caesar Salad	Turkey Chili	Greek Yogurt
4	Blueberry Pancakes	Quinoa Salad	Grilled Shrimp Skewers	Cheese and Crackers
5	Banana Nut Muffins	Tuna Salad	Ratatouille	Rice Cakes with Hummus
6	Greek Yogurt Parfait	Lentil Soup	Chicken Stir-Fry	Mixed Nuts
7	Vegetable Frittata	Minestrone Soup	Beef Stew	Carrot Sticks with Hummus
8	Strawberry Banana Smoothie	Black Bean Soup	Baked Cod	Cottage Cheese
9	Avocado Toast	Chicken Noodle Soup	Pork Tenderloin	Popcorn
10	Breakfast Quesadilla	Caprese Salad	Vegetable Stir-Fry	Sliced Cucumber with Lemon
11	Spinach and Mushroom Omelette	Egg Salad Sandwich	Stuffed Peppers	Fruit Salad

Day	Breakfast	Lunch	Dinner	Snacks
12	Whole Grain Waffles	Tomato Basil Soup	Turkey Meatballs	Edamame
13	Breakfast Casserole	Greek Chickpea Salad	Baked Chicken Parmesan	Pretzels
14	Yogurt and Berry Bowl	Vegetable Barley Soup	Lemon Garlic Tilapia	Roasted Chickpeas
15	Cinnamon Raisin French Toast	Chicken and Rice Soup	Beef and Broccoli	Yogurt Bark
16	Apple Cinnamon Oatmeal	Spinach and Lentil Salad	Mushroom Risotto	Peanut Butter Banana Bites
17	Blueberry Pancakes	Roasted Vegetable Wrap	Spinach and Feta Stuffed Chicken	Veggie Chips
18	Banana Nut Muffins	Beef and Barley Soup	Lentil Curry	Apple Slices with Peanut Butter
19	Greek Yogurt Parfait	Turkey and Avocado Wrap	Baked Salmon	Trail Mix
20	Vegetable Frittata	Greek Salad	Lemon Herb Chicken	Greek Yogurt

Meal Plan for Days 21-30

Day	Breakfast	Lunch	Dinner	Snacks
21	Strawberry Banana Smoothie	Chicken Caesar Salad	Turkey Chili	Cheese and Crackers
22	Avocado Toast	Quinoa Salad	Grilled Shrimp Skewers	Rice Cakes with Hummus
23	Breakfast Quesadilla	Tuna Salad	Ratatouille	Mixed Nuts

Day	Breakfast	Lunch	Dinner	Snacks
24	Spinach and Mushroom Omelette	Lentil Soup	Chicken Stir-Fry	Carrot Sticks with Hummus
25	Whole Grain Waffles	Minestrone Soup	Beef Stew	Cottage Cheese
26	Breakfast Casserole	Black Bean Soup	Baked Cod	Popcorn
27	Yogurt and Berry Bowl	Chicken Noodle Soup	Pork Tenderloin	Sliced Cucumber with Lemon
28	Cinnamon Raisin French Toast	Caprese Salad	Vegetable Stir-Fry	Fruit Salad
29	Apple Cinnamon Oatmeal	Egg Salad Sandwich	Stuffed Peppers	Edamame
30	Blueberry Pancakes	Tomato Basil Soup	Turkey Meatballs	Pretzels

Breakfast

Yogurt and Berry Bowl

Prep Time: 10 minutes | **Cook Time:** 0 minutes | **Servings:** 2

Ingredients:

- 1 cup plain low-fat yogurt
- 1 cup mixed berries (such as strawberries, blueberries, and raspberries), fresh or frozen
- 2 tablespoons chopped almonds, unsalted
- 1 tablespoon honey (optional)
- 1/4 teaspoon cinnamon (optional)

Instructions:

1. If using frozen berries, thaw them in the refrigerator overnight or microwave them until slightly softened.
2. In a bowl, divide the plain low-fat yogurt equally into two servings.
3. Top each portion of yogurt with mixed berries.
4. Sprinkle 1 tablespoon of chopped unsalted almonds over each bowl.
5. Drizzle honey (if using) evenly over the bowls.
6. Optionally, sprinkle a pinch of cinnamon over the top for added flavor.
7. Serve immediately and enjoy!

Nutritional Information (per serving):

- Carbs: 25g
- Sodium: 40mg
- Potassium: 250mg
- Phosphorus: 150mg
- Protein: 7g

Cinnamon Raisin French Toast

Prep Time: 10 minutes | **Cook Time:** 10 minutes | **Servings:** 2

Ingredients:

- 4 slices low-phosphorus bread
- 2 eggs
- 1/4 cup low-fat milk
- 1/2 teaspoon ground cinnamon
- 1/4 cup raisins
- 1 teaspoon unsalted butter or cooking spray
- Sugar-free syrup, for serving (optional)

Instructions:

1. In a shallow dish, whisk together 2 eggs, low-fat milk, and ground cinnamon until well combined.
2. Soak each slice of low-phosphorus bread in the egg mixture for about 30 seconds on each side, ensuring they are evenly coated.
3. Sprinkle raisins over the soaked bread slices.
4. In a non-stick skillet, melt unsalted butter over medium heat or coat with cooking spray.
5. Cook the soaked bread slices for about 3-4 minutes on each side until golden brown and cooked through.
6. Remove from the skillet and serve hot.
7. Optionally, serve with sugar-free syrup if desired.

Nutritional Information (per serving):

- Carbs: 25g
- Sodium: 100mg
- Potassium: 150mg
- Phosphorus: 100mg
- Protein: 9g

Amanda K. Sanders

Apple Cinnamon Oatmeal

Prep Time: 10 minutes | **Cook Time:** 20 minutes | **Servings:** 2

Ingredients:

- 1 cup rolled oats
- 2 cups water
- 1 medium apple, peeled, cored, and diced
- 1 teaspoon ground cinnamon
- 1 tablespoon honey (optional)
- 1/4 cup chopped walnuts (optional)
- 1/4 cup low-fat milk or almond milk (optional)

Instructions:

1. In a medium saucepan, bring 2 cups of water to a boil.
2. Add 1 cup of rolled oats to the boiling water. Reduce heat to medium-low and simmer for 10 minutes, stirring occasionally.
3. While the oats are cooking, peel, core, and dice the apple.
4. After 10 minutes, add the diced apple and 1 teaspoon of ground cinnamon to the oatmeal. Stir adequately to combine.
5. Continue to cook for an additional 5-7 minutes until the apples are tender and the oatmeal has reached your desired consistency.
6. If desired, sweeten the oatmeal with 1 tablespoon of honey, and add chopped walnuts for extra crunch.
7. Serve the oatmeal hot, optionally topped with a splash of low-fat milk or almond milk.

Nutritional Information (per serving):

- Carbs: 40g
- Sodium: 5mg
- Potassium: 180mg
- Phosphorus: 95mg
- Protein: 6g

Blueberry Pancakes

Prep Time: 10 minutes | **Cook Time:** 15 minutes | **Servings:** 2

Ingredients:

- 1 cup whole wheat flour
- 1 tablespoon baking powder
- 1 tablespoon granulated sugar
- 1/4 teaspoon salt
- 1 cup unsweetened almond milk or low-fat milk
- 1 large egg
- 1 tablespoon vegetable oil
- 1/2 cup fresh or frozen blueberries
- Cooking spray or additional oil for greasing the pan

Instructions:

1. In a mixing bowl, combine 1 cup whole wheat flour, 1 tablespoon baking powder, 1 tablespoon granulated sugar, and 1/4 teaspoon salt.
2. In a separate bowl, whisk together 1 cup unsweetened almond milk or low-fat milk, 1 large egg, and 1 tablespoon vegetable oil until well combined.
3. Gradually add the wet ingredients to the dry ingredients, stirring until just combined. Be careful not to overmix; it's okay if the batter is slightly lumpy.
4. Gently fold in 1/2 cup of fresh or frozen blueberries into the batter.
5. Heat a non-stick skillet or griddle over medium heat and lightly grease with cooking spray or additional oil.
6. Pour about 1/4 cup of batter onto the skillet for each pancake. Cook until bubbles form on the surface of the pancake and the edges look set, about 2-3 minutes.
7. Flip the pancakes and cook for an additional 1-2 minutes on the other side, or until golden brown and cooked through.
8. Repeat with the remaining batter, greasing the skillet as needed.
9. Serve the pancakes warm, optionally topped with additional blueberries and a drizzle of maple syrup.

Nutritional Information (per serving):

- Carbs: 39g
- Sodium: 280mg
- Potassium: 220mg
- Phosphorus: 200mg
- Protein: 7g

Banana Nut Muffins

Prep Time: 10 minutes | **Cook Time:** 20 minutes | **Servings:** 12

Ingredients:

- 1 1/2 cups whole wheat flour
- 1 teaspoon baking powder
- 1/2 teaspoon baking soda
- 1/4 teaspoon salt
- 3 ripe bananas, mashed
- 1/3 cup unsweetened applesauce
- 1/4 cup honey or maple syrup
- 1 large egg
- 1 teaspoon vanilla extract
- 1/2 cup chopped walnuts

Instructions:

1. Preheat the oven to 350°F (175°C). Grease a 12-cup muffin tin or line with paper liners.
2. In a large mixing bowl, combine 1 1/2 cups whole wheat flour, 1 teaspoon baking powder, 1/2 teaspoon baking soda, and 1/4 teaspoon salt.
3. In another bowl, mash 3 ripe bananas using a fork or potato masher.
4. Add 1/3 cup unsweetened applesauce, 1/4 cup honey or maple syrup, 1 large egg, and 1 teaspoon vanilla extract to the mashed bananas. Mix until well combined.
5. Pour the wet ingredients into the dry ingredients and stir until just combined. Do not overmix.
6. Gently fold in 1/2 cup of chopped walnuts into the batter.
7. Divide the batter evenly among the prepared muffin cups, filling each about 2/3 full.
8. Bake in the preheated oven for 18-20 minutes, or until a toothpick inserted into the center of a muffin comes out clean.
9. Allow the muffins to cool in the pan for 5 minutes before transferring them to a wire rack to cool completely.

Nutritional Information (per serving):

- Carbs: 23g
- Sodium: 100mg
- Potassium: 180mg
- Phosphorus: 90mg
- Protein: 3g

Greek Yogurt Parfait

Prep Time: 10 minutes | **Cook Time:** 0 minutes | **Servings:** 2

Ingredients:

- 1 cup low-fat Greek yogurt
- 1/2 cup fresh strawberries, diced
- 1/2 cup fresh blueberries
- 2 tablespoons chopped almonds or walnuts (optional)
- 2 tablespoons honey or maple syrup (optional)

Instructions:

1. In two serving glasses or bowls, layer 1/2 cup of low-fat Greek yogurt at the bottom of each.
2. Top the yogurt with 1/4 cup of diced fresh strawberries in each glass.
3. Add 1/4 cup of fresh blueberries on top of the strawberries in each glass.
4. Sprinkle 1 tablespoon of chopped almonds or walnuts on top of the berries in each glass if desired.
5. Drizzle 1 tablespoon of honey or maple syrup over each parfait if desired.
6. Serve immediately, or refrigerate until ready to serve.

Nutritional Information (per serving):

- Carbs: 25g
- Sodium: 50mg
- Potassium: 200mg
- Phosphorus: 90mg
- Protein: 12g

Vegetable Frittata

Prep Time: 10 minutes | **Cook Time:** 20 minutes | **Servings:** 4

Ingredients:

- 6 large eggs
- 1/4 cup low-fat milk
- 1/4 teaspoon salt
- 1/4 teaspoon black pepper
- 1 tablespoon olive oil
- 1/2 cup diced onion
- 1/2 cup diced bell pepper
- 1/2 cup diced zucchini
- 1/2 cup diced tomatoes
- 1/4 cup chopped fresh spinach
- 2 tablespoons grated Parmesan cheese (optional)

Instructions:

1. Preheat the oven to 350°F (175°C).
2. In a mixing bowl, whisk together 6 large eggs, 1/4 cup low-fat milk, 1/4 teaspoon salt, and 1/4 teaspoon black pepper until well combined. Set aside.
3. Heat 1 tablespoon of olive oil in an oven-safe skillet over medium heat.
4. Add 1/2 cup diced onion, 1/2 cup diced bell pepper, and 1/2 cup diced zucchini to the skillet. Cook until the vegetables are softened, about 5 minutes.
5. Add 1/2 cup diced tomatoes and 1/4 cup chopped fresh spinach to the skillet. Cook for an additional 2 minutes until the spinach wilts.
6. Pour the egg mixture over the cooked vegetables in the skillet. Stir gently to distribute the vegetables evenly.
7. Cook the frittata on the stovetop for 3-4 minutes, or until the edges begin to set.
8. Sprinkle 2 tablespoons of grated Parmesan cheese evenly over the top of the frittata, if desired.
9. Transfer the skillet to the preheated oven and bake for 10-12 minutes, or until the frittata is set in the center and lightly golden on top.
10. Take out the skillet from the oven and let the frittata cool for a few minutes before slicing and serving.

Nutritional Information (per serving):

- Carbs: 6g
- Sodium: 160mg
- Potassium: 210mg
- Phosphorus: 120mg
- Protein: 11g

Strawberry Banana Smoothie

Prep Time: 5 minutes | **Cook Time:** 0 minutes | **Servings:** 2

Ingredients:

- 1 ripe banana
- 1 cup fresh strawberries, hulled and halved
- 1 cup unsweetened almond milk or low-fat milk
- 1/2 cup low-fat Greek yogurt
- 1 tablespoon honey or maple syrup (optional)
- Ice cubes (optional)

Instructions:

1. Peel 1 ripe banana and cut it into chunks.
2. Hull and halve 1 cup of fresh strawberries.
3. In a blender, put in the banana chunks, halved strawberries, 1 cup of unsweetened almond milk or low-fat milk, and 1/2 cup of low-fat Greek yogurt.
4. If desired, add 1 tablespoon of honey or maple syrup for sweetness.
5. Optionally, add a handful of ice cubes to the blender to make the smoothie colder and thicker.
6. Blend all the ingredients until smooth and creamy, scraping down the sides of the blender as needed.
7. Once the smoothie reaches your desired consistency, pour it into glasses and serve immediately.

Nutritional Information (per serving):

- Carbs: 23g
- Sodium: 90mg
- Potassium: 300mg
- Phosphorus: 100mg
- Protein: 5g

Avocado Toast

Prep Time: 10 minutes | **Cook Time:** 0 minutes | **Servings:** 2

Ingredients:

- 2 slices whole wheat bread
- 1 ripe avocado
- 1 tablespoon lemon juice
- Salt, to taste
- Black pepper, to taste
- Red pepper flakes, for garnish (optional)
- Chopped fresh cilantro or parsley, for garnish (optional)

Instructions:

1. Toast 2 slices of whole wheat bread until golden brown.
2. Cut 1 ripe avocado in half, take out the pit, and scoop the flesh into a bowl.
3. Add 1 tablespoon of lemon juice to the avocado flesh to prevent browning.
4. Mash the avocado with a fork until smooth.
5. Season the mashed avocado with salt and black pepper to taste. Mix adequately.
6. Spread the mashed avocado evenly onto the toasted whole wheat bread slices.
7. Garnish with red pepper flakes and chopped fresh cilantro or parsley, if desired.
8. Serve the avocado toast immediately.

Nutritional Information (per serving):

- Carbs: 20g
- Sodium: 100mg
- Potassium: 450mg
- Phosphorus: 90mg
- Protein: 5g

Breakfast Quesadilla

Prep Time: 10 minutes | **Cook Time:** 10 minutes | **Servings:** 2

Ingredients:

- 2 large whole wheat tortillas
- 4 large eggs
- 1/4 cup low-fat milk
- Salt, to taste
- Black pepper, to taste
- 1/2 cup shredded low-sodium cheddar cheese
- 1/4 cup diced bell pepper
- 1/4 cup diced onion
- Cooking spray or olive oil

Instructions:

1. In a bowl, whisk together 4 large eggs, 1/4 cup low-fat milk, salt, and black pepper until well combined.
2. Heat a non-stick skillet over medium heat and spray with cooking spray or add a small amount of olive oil.
3. Pour the egg mixture into the skillet and cook, stirring occasionally, until the eggs are scrambled and cooked through. Remove from heat and set aside.
4. Wipe the skillet clean and return it to the heat.
5. Place 1 whole wheat tortilla in the skillet and sprinkle half of the shredded low-sodium cheddar cheese evenly over the tortilla.
6. Spread half of the scrambled eggs over the cheese.
7. Sprinkle half of the diced bell pepper and half of the diced onion over the eggs.
8. Top with the remaining shredded low-sodium cheddar cheese and place the second whole wheat tortilla on top.
9. Cook the quesadilla for 2-3 minutes on each side, or until the tortillas are golden brown and the cheese is melted.
10. Take out the quesadilla from the skillet and let it cool for a minute before slicing into wedges.
11. Repeat the process with the remaining ingredients to make the second quesadilla.
12. Serve the breakfast quesadillas hot.

Nutritional Information (per serving):

- Carbs: 30g
- Sodium: 180mg
- Potassium: 220mg
- Phosphorus: 130mg
- Protein: 17g

Amanda K. Sanders

Spinach and Mushroom Omelette

Prep Time: 10 minutes | **Cook Time:** 10 minutes | **Servings:** 2

Ingredients:

- 4 large eggs
- 1/4 cup low-fat milk
- Salt, to taste
- Black pepper, to taste
- 1 tablespoon olive oil
- 1 cup fresh spinach leaves
- 1/2 cup sliced mushrooms
- 1/4 cup diced onion
- 1/4 cup shredded low-sodium mozzarella cheese

Instructions:

1. In a bowl, whisk together 4 large eggs, 1/4 cup low-fat milk, salt, and black pepper until well combined.
2. Heat 1 tablespoon of olive oil in a non-stick skillet over medium heat.
3. Add 1 cup of fresh spinach leaves, 1/2 cup of sliced mushrooms, and 1/4 cup of diced onion to the skillet. Cook until the vegetables are tender, about 3-4 minutes.
4. Take out the cooked vegetables from the skillet and set aside.
5. Wipe the skillet clean and return it to the heat.
6. Pour the egg mixture into the skillet and tilt the pan to spread the eggs evenly.
7. Cook the eggs for 2-3 minutes, lifting the edges with a spatula to let the uncooked eggs flow underneath.
8. Once the eggs are mostly set, spread the cooked vegetables evenly over one half of the omelette.
9. Sprinkle 1/4 cup of shredded low-sodium mozzarella cheese over the vegetables.
10. Fold the other half of the omelette over the filling to form a half-moon shape.
11. Cook for another 2-3 minutes, or until the cheese is melted and the omelette is cooked through.
12. Carefully slide the omelette onto a plate and cut it in half.
13. Serve the spinach and mushroom omelette hot.

Nutritional Information (per serving):

- Carbs: 6g
- Sodium: 170mg
- Potassium: 320mg
- Phosphorus: 160mg
- Protein: 15g

Whole Grain Waffles

Prep Time: 10 minutes | **Cook Time:** 15 minutes | **Servings:** 4

Ingredients:

- 1 cup whole wheat flour
- 1/2 cup oat flour
- 2 teaspoons baking powder
- 1/4 teaspoon salt
- 1 1/4 cups unsweetened almond milk or low-fat milk
- 2 large eggs
- 2 tablespoons unsweetened applesauce
- 1 tablespoon honey or maple syrup (optional)
- Cooking spray or olive oil for greasing the waffle iron

Instructions:

1. In a large mixing bowl, whisk together 1 cup whole wheat flour, 1/2 cup oat flour, 2 teaspoons baking powder, and 1/4 teaspoon salt.
2. In a separate bowl, whisk together 1 1/4 cups unsweetened almond milk or low-fat milk, 2 large eggs, and 2 tablespoons unsweetened applesauce until well combined.
3. Gradually add the wet ingredients to the dry ingredients, stirring until just combined. Be careful not to overmix; it's okay if the batter is slightly lumpy.
4. If desired, sweeten the batter with 1 tablespoon of honey or maple syrup.
5. Preheat your waffle iron according to the manufacturer's instructions.
6. Once the waffle iron is ready, lightly grease it with cooking spray or olive oil.
7. Pour enough batter onto the center of the waffle iron to cover about two-thirds of the surface area.
8. Close the waffle iron and cook according to the manufacturer's instructions, or until the waffles are golden brown and crisp.
9. Carefully take out the waffles from the waffle iron and repeat with the remaining batter.
10. Serve the whole grain waffles hot, optionally topped with fresh fruit or a drizzle of maple syrup.

Nutritional Information (per serving):

- Carbs: 35g
- Sodium: 280mg
- Potassium: 160mg
- Phosphorus: 210mg
- Protein: 8g

Breakfast Casserole

Prep Time: 10 minutes | **Cook Time:** 20 minutes | **Servings:** 6

Ingredients:

- 6 large eggs
- 1 cup unsweetened almond milk or low-fat milk
- 4 slices whole wheat bread, cubed
- 1 cup diced cooked ham
- 1/2 cup diced bell pepper
- 1/2 cup diced onion
- 1/2 cup shredded low-sodium cheddar cheese
- Salt, to taste
- Black pepper, to taste
- Cooking spray or olive oil

Instructions:

1. Preheat your oven to 375°F (190°C).
2. In a large mixing bowl, whisk together 6 large eggs and 1 cup of unsweetened almond milk or low-fat milk until well combined.
3. Add 4 slices of whole wheat bread, cubed, to the egg mixture and stir to combine. Let it sit for a few minutes to allow the bread to soak up the liquid.
4. Stir in 1 cup of diced cooked ham, 1/2 cup of diced bell pepper, 1/2 cup of diced onion, and 1/2 cup of shredded low-sodium cheddar cheese. Season with salt and black pepper to taste.
5. Lightly grease a 9x13-inch baking dish with cooking spray or olive oil.
6. Pour the egg mixture into the prepared baking dish, spreading it out evenly.
7. Bake in the preheated oven for 20-25 minutes, or until the casserole is set in the center and lightly golden on top.
8. Take out the casserole from the oven and let it cool for a few minutes before slicing and serving.

Nutritional Information (per serving):

- Carbs: 15g
- Sodium: 280mg
- Potassium: 180mg
- Phosphorus: 150mg
- Protein: 14g

Lunch

Turkey and Avocado Wrap

Prep Time: 15 minutes | **Cook Time:** 15 minutes | **Servings:** 4

Ingredients:

- 1 lb thinly sliced turkey breast (cooked)
- 1 avocado, sliced
- 4 large whole grain tortillas
- 1 cup baby spinach leaves
- 1/2 cup diced tomatoes
- 1/4 cup sliced red onions
- 1/4 cup low-fat Greek yogurt
- 2 tablespoons chopped fresh cilantro
- 1 tablespoon lime juice
- Salt and pepper to taste

Nutritional Information (per serving):

- Carbs: 27g
- Sodium: 320mg
- Potassium: 400mg
- Phosphorus: 150mg
- Protein: 25g

Instructions:

1. In a small bowl, mix together the low-fat Greek yogurt, chopped cilantro, lime juice, salt, and pepper to make the avocado spread. Set aside.
2. Lay out the whole grain tortillas on a clean surface.
3. Spread the avocado mixture evenly onto each tortilla.
4. Layer thinly sliced turkey breast, avocado slices, baby spinach leaves, diced tomatoes, and sliced red onions onto each tortilla.
5. Roll up the tortillas tightly, tucking in the ends as you go, to form wraps.
6. Slice each wrap in half diagonally and serve immediately.

Greek Salad

Prep Time: 15 minutes | **Cook Time:** 0 minutes | **Servings:** 4

Ingredients:

- 4 cups chopped romaine lettuce
- 1 cup sliced cucumbers
- 1 cup diced tomatoes
- 1/2 cup sliced red onions
- 1/2 cup sliced black olives
- 1/4 cup crumbled feta cheese
- 2 tablespoons extra virgin olive oil
- 2 tablespoons red wine vinegar
- 1 teaspoon dried oregano
- Salt and pepper to taste

Nutritional Information (per serving):

- Carbs: 9g
- Sodium: 200mg
- Potassium: 250mg
- Phosphorus: 100mg
- Protein: 3g

Instructions:

1. In a large salad bowl, put in the chopped romaine lettuce, sliced cucumbers, diced tomatoes, sliced red onions, sliced black olives, and crumbled feta cheese.
2. In a small bowl, whisk together the extra virgin olive oil, red wine vinegar, dried oregano, salt, and pepper to make the dressing.
3. Drizzle the dressing over the salad and toss gently to coat all ingredients evenly.

Chicken Caesar Salad

Prep Time: 15 minutes | **Cook Time:** 15 minutes | **Servings:** 4

Ingredients:

- 2 boneless, skinless chicken breasts
- 4 cups chopped romaine lettuce
- 1/4 cup grated Parmesan cheese
- 1/4 cup croutons (optional; use low sodium if desired)
- 1/4 cup Caesar dressing (low sodium)
- 1 tablespoon olive oil
- Salt and pepper to taste

Nutritional Information (per serving):

1. Carbs: 5g
2. Sodium: 220mg
3. Potassium: 200mg
4. Phosphorus: 100mg
5. Protein: 25g

Instructions:

1. Season the chicken breasts with salt and pepper.
2. In a skillet over medium heat, add olive oil. Cook the chicken breasts for about 6-8 minutes on each side, or until cooked through. Remove from heat and let them rest for a few minutes before slicing.
3. Meanwhile, in a large salad bowl, put in the chopped romaine lettuce, grated Parmesan cheese, and croutons (if using).
4. Slice the cooked chicken breasts and add them to the salad.
5. Drizzle Caesar dressing over the salad and toss gently to coat all ingredients evenly.

Quinoa Salad

Prep Time: 15 minutes | **Cook Time:** 15 minutes | **Servings:** 4

Ingredients:

- 1 cup quinoa
- 2 cups low sodium vegetable broth
- 1 cup diced cucumbers
- 1 cup diced tomatoes
- 1/2 cup diced red bell peppers
- 1/4 cup chopped fresh parsley
- 1/4 cup chopped fresh mint
- 2 tablespoons extra virgin olive oil
- 2 tablespoons lemon juice
- Salt and pepper to taste

Nutritional Information (per serving):

- Carbs: 30g
- Sodium: 50mg
- Potassium: 250mg
- Phosphorus: 100mg
- Protein: 6g

Instructions:

1. Rinse the quinoa under cold water using a fine-mesh sieve.
2. In a medium saucepan, put in the rinsed quinoa and low sodium vegetable broth. Bring to a boil over medium-high heat.
3. Reduce the heat to low, cover, and simmer for 15 minutes, or until the quinoa is cooked and the liquid is absorbed. Remove from heat and let it cool.
4. In a large salad bowl, put in the cooked quinoa, diced cucumbers, diced tomatoes, diced red bell peppers, chopped fresh parsley, and chopped fresh mint.
5. In a small bowl, whisk together the extra virgin olive oil, lemon juice, salt, and pepper to make the dressing.
6. Drizzle the dressing over the salad and toss gently to coat all ingredients evenly.

Tuna Salad

Prep Time: 15 minutes | **Cook Time:** 0 minutes | **Servings:** 4

Ingredients:

- 2 cans (5 oz each) low sodium tuna, drained
- 1/2 cup diced celery
- 1/4 cup diced red onions
- 1/4 cup diced pickles (use low sodium pickles if available)
- 2 tablespoons low-fat mayonnaise
- 1 tablespoon lemon juice
- 1 teaspoon Dijon mustard
- Salt and pepper to taste
- 4 cups mixed salad greens

Nutritional Information (per serving):

- Carbs: 5g
- Sodium: 150mg
- Potassium: 150mg
- Phosphorus: 100mg
- Protein: 15g

Instructions:

1. In a large mixing bowl, put in the drained low sodium tuna, diced celery, diced red onions, and diced pickles.
2. In a small bowl, mix together the low-fat mayonnaise, lemon juice, Dijon mustard, salt, and pepper to make the dressing.
3. Pour the dressing over the tuna mixture and toss until well combined.
4. Serve the tuna salad over mixed salad greens.

Lentil Soup

Prep Time: 10 minutes | **Cook Time:** 20 minutes | **Servings:** 4

Ingredients:

- 1 cup dried green lentils, rinsed
- 4 cups low sodium vegetable broth
- 1 cup diced carrots
- 1 cup diced celery
- 1/2 cup diced onions
- 2 cloves garlic, minced
- 1 teaspoon dried thyme
- 1 bay leaf
- Salt and pepper to taste
- Chopped fresh parsley for garnish (optional)

Nutritional Information (per serving):

- Carbs: 30g
- Sodium: 150mg
- Potassium: 400mg
- Phosphorus: 150mg
- Protein: 15g

Instructions:

1. In a large pot, put in the rinsed green lentils, low sodium vegetable broth, diced carrots, diced celery, diced onions, minced garlic, dried thyme, and bay leaf.
2. Bring the mixture to a boil over medium-high heat.
3. Reduce the heat to low, cover, and simmer for 15-20 minutes, or until the lentils and vegetables are tender.
4. Season with salt and pepper to taste.
5. Take out the bay leaf before serving.
6. Garnish with chopped fresh parsley if desired.

Minestrone Soup

Prep Time: 10 minutes | **Cook Time:** 20 minutes | **Servings:** 4

Ingredients:

- 4 cups low sodium vegetable broth
- 1 can (14.5 oz) low sodium diced tomatoes
- 1 cup diced carrots
- 1 cup diced celery
- 1 cup diced zucchini
- 1/2 cup diced onions
- 2 cloves garlic, minced
- 1 teaspoon dried oregano
- 1 teaspoon dried basil
- 1/2 cup small pasta (such as ditalini or elbow)
- Salt and pepper to taste
- Chopped fresh parsley for garnish (optional)

Nutritional Information (per serving):

- Carbs: 25g
- Sodium: 200mg
- Potassium: 300mg
- Phosphorus: 100mg
- Protein: 5g

Instructions:

1. In a large pot, put in the low sodium vegetable broth, low sodium diced tomatoes, diced carrots, diced celery, diced zucchini, diced onions, minced garlic, dried oregano, and dried basil.
2. Bring the mixture to a boil over medium-high heat.
3. Reduce the heat to low and simmer for 10 minutes.
4. Add the small pasta to the pot and continue to simmer for another 8-10 minutes, or until the pasta is cooked and the vegetables are tender.
5. Season with salt and pepper to taste.
6. Remove from heat and serve hot.
7. Garnish with chopped fresh parsley if desired.

Black Bean Soup

Prep Time: 10 minutes | **Cook Time:** 20 minutes | **Servings:** 4

Ingredients:

- 2 cans (15 oz each) low sodium black beans, drained and rinsed
- 4 cups low sodium vegetable broth
- 1 cup diced onions
- 1 cup diced bell peppers (any color)
- 2 cloves garlic, minced
- 1 teaspoon ground cumin
- 1/2 teaspoon chili powder
- 1/4 teaspoon smoked paprika
- Salt and pepper to taste
- Chopped fresh cilantro for garnish (optional)
- Low-fat Greek yogurt or sour cream for garnish (optional)

Nutritional Information (per serving):

- Carbs: 30g
- Sodium: 200mg
- Potassium: 400mg
- Phosphorus: 150mg
- Protein: 10g

Instructions:

1. In a large pot, put in the drained and rinsed low sodium black beans, low sodium vegetable broth, diced onions, diced bell peppers, minced garlic, ground cumin, chili powder, and smoked paprika.
2. Bring the mixture to a boil over medium-high heat.
3. Reduce the heat to low and simmer for 15-20 minutes, stirring occasionally.
4. Using an immersion blender or regular blender, blend the soup until smooth and creamy. Be careful when blending hot liquids.
5. Season with salt and pepper to taste.
6. Serve hot, garnished with chopped fresh cilantro and a dollop of low-fat Greek yogurt or sour cream if desired.

Chicken Noodle Soup

Prep Time: 10 minutes | **Cook Time:** 20 minutes | **Servings:** 4

Ingredients:

- 4 cups low sodium chicken broth
- 2 cups water
- 2 boneless, skinless chicken breasts, diced
- 1 cup sliced carrots
- 1 cup diced celery
- 1/2 cup diced onions
- 2 cloves garlic, minced
- 1 teaspoon dried thyme
- 1 teaspoon dried parsley
- 1/2 teaspoon black pepper
- 2 cups uncooked egg noodles
- Salt to taste
- Chopped fresh parsley for garnish (optional)

Nutritional Information (per serving):

- Carbs: 20g
- Sodium: 150mg
- Potassium: 200mg
- Phosphorus: 100mg
- Protein: 15g

Instructions:

1. In a large pot, put in the low sodium chicken broth, water, diced boneless, skinless chicken breasts, sliced carrots, diced celery, diced onions, minced garlic, dried thyme, dried parsley, and black pepper.
2. Bring the mixture to a boil over medium-high heat.
3. Reduce the heat to low and simmer for 15 minutes, or until the chicken is cooked through and the vegetables are tender.
4. Add the uncooked egg noodles to the pot and continue to simmer for another 5-7 minutes, or until the noodles are cooked.
5. Season with salt to taste.
6. Remove from heat and serve hot.
7. Garnish with chopped fresh parsley if desired.

Caprese Salad

Prep Time: 10 minutes | **Cook Time:** 0 minutes | **Servings:** 4

Ingredients:

- 2 large tomatoes, sliced
- 1 ball fresh mozzarella cheese, sliced
- 1/4 cup fresh basil leaves
- 2 tablespoons extra virgin olive oil
- 1 tablespoon balsamic vinegar
- Salt and pepper to taste

Nutritional Information (per serving):

- Carbs: 5g
- Sodium: 100mg
- Potassium: 200mg
- Phosphorus: 50mg
- Protein: 5g

Instructions:

1. Arrange the sliced tomatoes and fresh mozzarella cheese alternately on a serving platter.
2. Tuck fresh basil leaves between the tomato and cheese slices.
3. Drizzle extra virgin olive oil and balsamic vinegar over the salad.
4. Season with salt and pepper to taste.

Egg Salad Sandwich

Prep Time: 10 minutes | **Cook Time:** 10 minutes | **Servings:** 4

Ingredients:

- 6 large eggs
- 1/4 cup low-fat mayonnaise
- 1 tablespoon Dijon mustard
- 2 tablespoons finely chopped celery
- 2 tablespoons finely chopped green onions
- Salt and pepper to taste
- 8 slices whole wheat bread
- Lettuce leaves for serving (optional)
- Tomato slices for serving (optional)

Nutritional Information (per serving):

- Carbs: 20g
- Sodium: 150mg
- Potassium: 150mg
- Phosphorus: 100mg
- Protein: 10g

Instructions:

1. Place the eggs in a saucepan and cover them with water. Bring the water to a boil over medium-high heat.
2. Once boiling, cover the saucepan and remove it from heat. Let the eggs sit in the hot water for 10 minutes.
3. Drain the hot water and fill the saucepan with cold water and ice cubes to cool the eggs quickly.
4. Once cooled, peel the eggs and chop them finely.
5. In a mixing bowl, put in the chopped hard-boiled eggs, low-fat mayonnaise, Dijon mustard, finely chopped celery, and finely chopped green onions. Mix adequately to combine.
6. Season the egg salad with salt and pepper to taste.
7. Toast the slices of whole wheat bread.
8. Divide the egg salad evenly among 4 slices of toasted bread.
9. Top each sandwich with another slice of toasted bread.
10. Serve the egg salad sandwiches with lettuce leaves and tomato slices if desired.

Tomato Basil Soup

Prep Time: 10 minutes | **Cook Time:** 20 minutes | **Servings:** 4

Ingredients:

- 2 cans (14.5 oz each) no salt added diced tomatoes
- 2 cups low sodium vegetable broth
- 1/2 cup diced onions
- 2 cloves garlic, minced
- 1/4 cup chopped fresh basil leaves
- 1 tablespoon olive oil
- Salt and pepper to taste
- Optional: 1/4 cup low-fat Greek yogurt or sour cream for garnish

Nutritional Information (per serving):

- Carbs: 15g
- Sodium: 200mg
- Potassium: 300mg
- Phosphorus: 50mg
- Protein: 3g

Instructions:

1. In a large pot, heat the olive oil over medium heat.
2. Add the diced onions and minced garlic to the pot. Cook until the onions are translucent and fragrant, about 3-4 minutes.
3. Add the no salt added diced tomatoes (with their juices) to the pot.
4. Pour in the low sodium vegetable broth.
5. Bring the mixture to a simmer and cook for 15 minutes.
6. Using an immersion blender or regular blender, blend the soup until smooth.
7. Stir in the chopped fresh basil leaves and simmer for an additional 5 minutes.
8. Season the soup with salt and pepper to taste.
9. Serve hot, optionally garnished with a dollop of low-fat Greek yogurt or sour cream.

Greek Chickpea Salad

Prep Time: 10 minutes | **Cook Time:** 0 minutes | **Servings:** 4

Ingredients:

- 2 cans (15 oz each) low sodium chickpeas, drained and rinsed
- 1 cup diced cucumbers
- 1 cup halved cherry tomatoes
- 1/2 cup diced red onions
- 1/4 cup chopped fresh parsley
- 1/4 cup crumbled feta cheese
- 2 tablespoons extra virgin olive oil
- 2 tablespoons lemon juice
- 1 teaspoon dried oregano
- Salt and pepper to taste

Nutritional Information (per serving):

- Carbs: 30g
- Sodium: 150mg
- Potassium: 250mg
- Phosphorus: 100mg
- Protein: 10g

Instructions:

1. In a large mixing bowl, put in the drained and rinsed low sodium chickpeas, diced cucumbers, halved cherry tomatoes, diced red onions, chopped fresh parsley, and crumbled feta cheese.
2. In a small bowl, whisk together the extra virgin olive oil, lemon juice, dried oregano, salt, and pepper to make the dressing.
3. Pour the dressing over the salad and toss gently to coat all ingredients evenly.

Vegetable Barley Soup

Prep Time: 10 minutes | **Cook Time:** 20 minutes | **Servings:** 4

Ingredients:

- 4 cups low sodium vegetable broth
- 2 cups water
- 1/2 cup pearl barley
- 1 cup diced carrots
- 1 cup diced celery
- 1 cup diced onions
- 2 cloves garlic, minced
- 1 teaspoon dried thyme
- 1 bay leaf
- Salt and pepper to taste
- Chopped fresh parsley for garnish (optional)

Nutritional Information (per serving):

- Carbs: 30g
- Sodium: 150mg
- Potassium: 250mg
- Phosphorus: 100mg
- Protein: 5g

Instructions:

1. In a large pot, put in the low sodium vegetable broth, water, pearl barley, diced carrots, diced celery, diced onions, minced garlic, dried thyme, and bay leaf.
2. Bring the mixture to a boil over medium-high heat.
3. Reduce the heat to low, cover, and simmer for 15-20 minutes, or until the barley and vegetables are tender.
4. Take out the bay leaf from the soup.
5. Season with salt and pepper to taste.
6. Serve hot, garnished with chopped fresh parsley if desired.

Chicken and Rice Soup

Prep Time: 10 minutes | **Cook Time:** 20 minutes | **Servings:** 4

Ingredients:

- 4 cups low sodium chicken broth
- 2 cups water
- 2 boneless, skinless chicken breasts, diced
- 1/2 cup diced carrots
- 1/2 cup diced celery
- 1/2 cup diced onions
- 1/2 cup uncooked white rice
- 2 cloves garlic, minced
- 1 teaspoon dried thyme
- Salt and pepper to taste
- Chopped fresh parsley for garnish (optional)

Nutritional Information (per serving):

- Carbs: 20g
- Sodium: 150mg
- Potassium: 200mg
- Phosphorus: 100mg
- Protein: 15g

Instructions:

1. In a large pot, put in the low sodium chicken broth, water, diced boneless, skinless chicken breasts, diced carrots, diced celery, diced onions, uncooked white rice, minced garlic, and dried thyme.
2. Bring the mixture to a boil over medium-high heat.
3. Reduce the heat to low and simmer for 15-20 minutes, or until the chicken is cooked through, the rice is tender, and the vegetables are soft.
4. Season with salt and pepper to taste.
5. Serve hot, garnished with chopped fresh parsley if desired.

Spinach and Lentil Salad

Prep Time: 15 minutes | **Cook Time:** 15 minutes | **Servings:** 4

Ingredients:

- 1 cup dried green lentils, rinsed
- 4 cups fresh spinach leaves, chopped
- 1/2 cup diced red bell pepper
- 1/4 cup diced red onion
- 1/4 cup crumbled feta cheese
- 2 tablespoons extra virgin olive oil
- 2 tablespoons balsamic vinegar
- 1 teaspoon Dijon mustard
- Salt and pepper to taste

Nutritional Information (per serving):

- Carbs: 30g
- Sodium: 100mg
- Potassium: 300mg
- Phosphorus: 100mg
- Protein: 10g

Instructions:

1. In a medium saucepan, put in the rinsed green lentils with enough water to cover them. Bring to a boil over medium-high heat.
2. Reduce the heat to low and simmer for 15 minutes, or until the lentils are tender but still firm. Drain any excess water and let the lentils cool.
3. In a large salad bowl, put in the chopped fresh spinach leaves, diced red bell pepper, diced red onion, crumbled feta cheese, and cooked green lentils.
4. In a small bowl, whisk together the extra virgin olive oil, balsamic vinegar, Dijon mustard, salt, and pepper to make the dressing.
5. Pour the dressing over the salad and toss gently to coat all ingredients evenly.

Roasted Vegetable Wrap

Prep Time: 10 minutes | **Cook Time:** 20 minutes | **Servings:** 4

Ingredients:

- 2 cups mixed vegetables (such as bell peppers, zucchini, and onions), sliced
- 2 tablespoons olive oil
- Salt and pepper to taste
- 4 whole wheat tortillas
- 1/2 cup hummus
- 1 cup fresh spinach leaves

Nutritional Information (per serving):

- Carbs: 30g
- Sodium: 150mg
- Potassium: 200mg
- Phosphorus: 100mg
- Protein: 5g

Instructions:

1. Preheat your oven to 400°F (200°C).
2. Place the sliced mixed vegetables on a baking sheet. Drizzle with olive oil and season with salt and pepper to taste. Toss to coat evenly.
3. Roast the vegetables in the preheated oven for 15-20 minutes, or until they are tender and slightly browned.
4. While the vegetables are roasting, warm the whole wheat tortillas in a dry skillet over medium heat for about 1 minute on each side.
5. Spread 2 tablespoons of hummus onto each tortilla.
6. Top each tortilla with a quarter of the roasted vegetables and a handful of fresh spinach leaves.
7. Roll up the tortillas tightly, folding in the sides as you go, to form wraps.
8. Slice each wrap in half diagonally before serving, if desired.

Beef and Barley Soup

Prep Time: 10 minutes | **Cook Time:** 20 minutes | **Servings:** 4

Ingredients:

- 1/2 pound lean beef, diced
- 1/2 cup pearl barley
- 4 cups low sodium beef broth
- 2 cups water
- 1 cup diced carrots
- 1 cup diced celery
- 1/2 cup diced onions
- 2 cloves garlic, minced
- 1 teaspoon dried thyme
- Salt and pepper to taste
- Chopped fresh parsley for garnish (optional)

Nutritional Information (per serving):

- Carbs: 20g
- Sodium: 200mg
- Potassium: 250mg
- Phosphorus: 100mg
- Protein: 15g

Instructions:

1. In a large pot, brown the diced lean beef over medium heat until cooked through.
2. Add the pearl barley, low sodium beef broth, water, diced carrots, diced celery, diced onions, minced garlic, and dried thyme to the pot with the cooked beef.
3. Bring the mixture to a boil over medium-high heat.
4. Reduce the heat to low and simmer for 15-20 minutes, or until the barley and vegetables are tender.
5. Season with salt and pepper to taste.
6. Serve hot, garnished with chopped fresh parsley if desired.

Dinner

Baked Salmon

Prep Time: 10 minutes | **Cook Time:** 20 minutes | **Servings:** 4

Ingredients:

- 4 salmon fillets (6 ounces each)
- 2 tablespoons olive oil
- 2 cloves garlic, minced
- 1 tablespoon lemon juice
- 1 teaspoon dried dill
- Salt and pepper to taste

Instructions:

1. Preheat your oven to 400°F (200°C).
2. Place the salmon fillets on a baking sheet lined with parchment paper.
3. In a small bowl, mix together the olive oil, minced garlic, lemon juice, dried dill, salt, and pepper.
4. Brush the mixture over the salmon fillets, ensuring they are evenly coated.
5. Bake the salmon in the preheated oven for 15-20 minutes, or until the salmon is cooked through and flakes easily with a fork.
6. Once baked, take out the salmon from the oven and let it rest for a few minutes before serving.

Nutritional Information (per serving):

- Carbs: 0g
- Sodium: 90mg
- Potassium: 380mg
- Phosphorus: 200mg
- Protein: 34g

Lemon Herb Chicken

Prep Time: 10 minutes | **Cook Time:** 20 minutes | **Servings:** 4

Ingredients:

- 4 boneless, skinless chicken breasts
- 2 tablespoons olive oil
- 2 cloves garlic, minced
- 2 tablespoons fresh lemon juice
- 1 tablespoon chopped fresh parsley
- 1 teaspoon dried oregano
- Salt and pepper to taste

Instructions:

1. Preheat a skillet over medium-high heat.
2. Season the chicken breasts with salt and pepper on both sides.
3. Add olive oil to the skillet, then add the chicken breasts.
4. Cook the chicken for about 6-8 minutes on each side, or until cooked through and no longer pink in the center.
5. In a small bowl, mix together the minced garlic, fresh lemon juice, chopped fresh parsley, and dried oregano.
6. Pour the lemon herb mixture over the cooked chicken breasts in the skillet.
7. Allow the chicken to simmer in the lemon herb sauce for an additional 2-3 minutes.
8. Serve the chicken breasts with the lemon herb sauce spooned over the top.

Nutritional Information (per serving):

- Carbs: 1g
- Sodium: 70mg
- Potassium: 300mg
- Phosphorus: 200mg
- Protein: 26g

Turkey Chili

Prep Time: 10 minutes | **Cook Time:** 20 minutes | **Servings:** 4

Ingredients:

- 1 pound ground turkey
- 1 tablespoon olive oil
- 1 onion, diced
- 2 cloves garlic, minced
- 1 bell pepper, diced
- 1 can (14.5 ounces) low-sodium diced tomatoes
- 1 can (15 ounces) low-sodium kidney beans, drained and rinsed
- 1 tablespoon chili powder
- 1 teaspoon ground cumin
- 1/2 teaspoon paprika
- Salt and pepper to taste

Instructions:

1. In a large skillet, heat olive oil over medium heat.
2. Add diced onion and minced garlic to the skillet. Sauté until onion is translucent.
3. Add ground turkey to the skillet and cook until browned, breaking it up with a spoon.
4. Stir in diced bell pepper, low-sodium diced tomatoes, and low-sodium kidney beans.
5. Add chili powder, ground cumin, paprika, salt, and pepper to the skillet. Stir to combine.
6. Let the chili simmer for about 15-20 minutes, stirring occasionally, until flavors are well combined and the chili is heated through.

Nutritional Information (per serving):

- Carbs: 20g
- Sodium: 220mg
- Potassium: 380mg
- Phosphorus: 150mg
- Protein: 22g

Grilled Shrimp Skewers

Prep Time: 15 minutes | **Cook Time:** 10 minutes | **Servings:** 4

Ingredients:

- 1 pound large shrimp, peeled and deveined
- 2 tablespoons olive oil
- 2 cloves garlic, minced
- 1 tablespoon fresh lemon juice
- 1 teaspoon dried oregano
- Salt and pepper to taste

Instructions:

1. Preheat your grill to medium-high heat.
2. In a bowl, combine olive oil, minced garlic, fresh lemon juice, dried oregano, salt, and pepper.
3. Add the peeled and deveined shrimp to the bowl and toss to coat them evenly with the marinade.
4. Thread the shrimp onto skewers, dividing them evenly.
5. Place the shrimp skewers on the preheated grill and cook for 2-3 minutes on each side, or until the shrimp are pink and opaque.
6. Take out the shrimp skewers from the grill and serve immediately.

Nutritional Information (per serving):

- Carbs: 1g
- Sodium: 110mg
- Potassium: 210mg
- Phosphorus: 170mg
- Protein: 23g

Ratatouille

Prep Time: 10 minutes | **Cook Time:** 20 minutes | **Servings:** 4

Ingredients:

- 1 small eggplant, diced
- 1 small zucchini, diced
- 1 small yellow squash, diced
- 1 red bell pepper, diced
- 1 onion, diced
- 2 cloves garlic, minced
- 2 tablespoons olive oil
- 1 can (14.5 ounces) low-sodium diced tomatoes
- 1 teaspoon dried thyme
- 1 teaspoon dried oregano
- Salt and pepper to taste

Instructions:

1. In a large skillet, heat olive oil over medium heat.
2. Add diced onion and minced garlic to the skillet. Sauté until onion is translucent.
3. Add diced eggplant, zucchini, yellow squash, and red bell pepper to the skillet. Cook for 5-7 minutes, or until vegetables are slightly softened.
4. Stir in low-sodium diced tomatoes, dried thyme, dried oregano, salt, and pepper.
5. Let the ratatouille simmer for another 10 minutes, stirring occasionally, until vegetables are tender.
6. Serve the ratatouille hot as a side dish or over cooked rice or pasta.

Nutritional Information (per serving):

- Carbs: 14g
- Sodium: 120mg
- Potassium: 420mg
- Phosphorus: 70mg
- Protein: 3g

Chicken Stir-Fry

Prep Time: 15 minutes | **Cook Time:** 15 minutes | **Servings:** 4

Ingredients:

- 1 pound boneless, skinless chicken breasts, sliced into thin strips
- 2 tablespoons low-sodium soy sauce
- 1 tablespoon olive oil
- 2 cloves garlic, minced
- 1 teaspoon grated fresh ginger
- 1 red bell pepper, sliced
- 1 green bell pepper, sliced
- 1 cup sliced mushrooms
- 1 cup snap peas
- 1 small onion, sliced
- Salt and pepper to taste

Instructions:

1. In a bowl, marinate the sliced chicken breasts with low-sodium soy sauce. Set aside for 10 minutes.
2. Heat olive oil in a large skillet or wok over medium-high heat.
3. Add minced garlic and grated fresh ginger to the skillet. Sauté for about 1 minute until fragrant.
4. Add the marinated chicken strips to the skillet. Cook for 5-6 minutes, or until chicken is no longer pink.
5. Add sliced red bell pepper, green bell pepper, mushrooms, snap peas, and sliced onion to the skillet. Stir-fry for another 4-5 minutes, or until vegetables are tender-crisp.
6. Season with salt and pepper to taste.
7. Serve the chicken stir-fry hot over cooked rice or noodles.

Nutritional Information (per serving):

- Carbs: 9g
- Sodium: 180mg
- Potassium: 340mg
- Phosphorus: 130mg
- Protein: 28g

Beef Stew

Prep Time: 10 minutes | **Cook Time:** 20 minutes | **Servings:** 4

Ingredients:

- 1 pound beef stew meat, cut into small pieces
- 2 tablespoons olive oil
- 1 onion, diced
- 2 cloves garlic, minced
- 2 carrots, sliced
- 2 celery stalks, sliced
- 2 cups low-sodium beef broth
- 1 tablespoon tomato paste
- 1 teaspoon dried thyme
- 1 teaspoon dried rosemary
- Salt and pepper to taste

Instructions:

1. In a large pot, heat olive oil over medium heat.
2. Add diced onion and minced garlic to the pot. Sauté until onion is translucent.
3. Add beef stew meat to the pot. Cook until browned on all sides.
4. Stir in sliced carrots and celery.
5. Add low-sodium beef broth, tomato paste, dried thyme, dried rosemary, salt, and pepper to the pot. Bring to a simmer.
6. Let the stew simmer for about 15-20 minutes, or until the beef is tender and the vegetables are cooked through.

Nutritional Information (per serving):

1. Carbs: 7g
2. Sodium: 130mg
3. Potassium: 300mg
4. Phosphorus: 160mg
5. Protein: 22g

Baked Cod

Prep Time: 10 minutes | **Cook Time:** 15 minutes | **Servings:** 4

Ingredients:

- 4 cod fillets (6 ounces each)
- 2 tablespoons olive oil
- 2 cloves garlic, minced
- 1 tablespoon fresh lemon juice
- 1 teaspoon dried parsley
- Salt and pepper to taste

Instructions:

1. Preheat your oven to 400°F (200°C).
2. Place the cod fillets on a baking sheet lined with parchment paper.
3. In a small bowl, mix together the olive oil, minced garlic, fresh lemon juice, dried parsley, salt, and pepper.
4. Brush the mixture over the cod fillets, ensuring they are evenly coated.
5. Bake the cod in the preheated oven for 12-15 minutes, or until the fish is opaque and flakes easily with a fork.
6. Once baked, take out the cod from the oven and let it rest for a few minutes before serving.

Nutritional Information (per serving):

- Carbs: 0g
- Sodium: 80mg
- Potassium: 350mg
- Phosphorus: 180mg
- Protein: 34g

Pork Tenderloin

Prep Time: 10 minutes | **Cook Time:** 20 minutes | **Servings:** 4

Ingredients:

- 1 pound pork tenderloin
- 2 tablespoons olive oil
- 2 cloves garlic, minced
- 1 tablespoon balsamic vinegar
- 1 teaspoon dried rosemary
- Salt and pepper to taste

Instructions:

1. Preheat your oven to 400°F (200°C).
2. In a small bowl, mix together the olive oil, minced garlic, balsamic vinegar, dried rosemary, salt, and pepper.
3. Place the pork tenderloin in a baking dish and pour the marinade over it, ensuring it's evenly coated.
4. Bake the pork tenderloin in the preheated oven for 20-25 minutes, or until the internal temperature reaches 145°F (63°C) when measured with a meat thermometer.
5. Once baked, take out the pork tenderloin from the oven and let it rest for a few minutes before slicing.

Nutritional Information (per serving):

- Carbs: 0g
- Sodium: 70mg
- Potassium: 280mg
- Phosphorus: 220mg
- Protein: 26g

Vegetable Stir-Fry

Prep Time: 10 minutes | **Cook Time:** 10 minutes | **Servings:** 4

Ingredients:

- 1 tablespoon olive oil
- 2 cloves garlic, minced
- 1 onion, sliced
- 1 bell pepper, sliced
- 2 carrots, julienned
- 1 cup broccoli florets
- 1 cup snap peas
- 2 tablespoons low-sodium soy sauce
- 1 tablespoon rice vinegar
- 1 teaspoon grated fresh ginger
- Salt and pepper to taste

Instructions:

1. Heat olive oil in a large skillet or wok over medium-high heat.
2. Add minced garlic to the skillet and sauté for about 1 minute until fragrant.
3. Add sliced onion, sliced bell pepper, julienned carrots, broccoli florets, and snap peas to the skillet. Stir-fry for 4-5 minutes, or until vegetables are tender-crisp.
4. In a small bowl, mix together low-sodium soy sauce, rice vinegar, and grated fresh ginger.
5. Pour the sauce over the vegetables in the skillet and toss to coat evenly.
6. Season with salt and pepper to taste.
7. Cook for another 1-2 minutes, stirring occasionally, until the sauce is heated through.
8. Serve the vegetable stir-fry hot as a side dish or over cooked rice or noodles.

Nutritional Information (per serving):

- Carbs: 12g
- Sodium: 150mg
- Potassium: 300mg
- Phosphorus: 60mg
- Protein: 3g

Stuffed Peppers

Prep Time: 10 minutes | **Cook Time:** 20 minutes | **Servings:** 4

Ingredients:

- 4 large bell peppers
- 1 cup cooked quinoa
- 1 can (14.5 ounces) low-sodium diced tomatoes, drained
- 1 cup diced zucchini
- 1 cup diced mushrooms
- 1/2 cup diced onion
- 2 cloves garlic, minced
- 1 teaspoon dried oregano
- 1 teaspoon dried basil
- Salt and pepper to taste

Instructions:

1. Preheat your oven to 375°F (190°C).
2. Cut the tops off the bell peppers and take out the seeds and membranes from inside.
3. In a large bowl, mix together cooked quinoa, drained low-sodium diced tomatoes, diced zucchini, diced mushrooms, diced onion, minced garlic, dried oregano, dried basil, salt, and pepper.
4. Stuff each bell pepper with the quinoa and vegetable mixture, pressing it down gently.
5. Place the stuffed peppers in a baking dish and cover the dish with foil.
6. Bake in the preheated oven for 20-25 minutes, or until the peppers are tender.
7. Take out the foil and bake for an additional 5 minutes to slightly brown the tops of the peppers.
8. Serve the stuffed peppers hot.

Nutritional Information (per serving):

- Carbs: 22g
- Sodium: 70mg
- Potassium: 500mg
- Phosphorus: 90mg
- Protein: 5g

Turkey Meatballs

Prep Time: 10 minutes | **Cook Time:** 20 minutes | **Servings:** 4

Ingredients:

- 1 pound ground turkey
- 1/4 cup breadcrumbs
- 1/4 cup grated Parmesan cheese
- 1 egg
- 2 cloves garlic, minced
- 1 tablespoon chopped fresh parsley
- 1/2 teaspoon dried oregano
- Salt and pepper to taste
- Olive oil, for cooking

Instructions:

1. Preheat your oven to 400°F (200°C).
2. In a large bowl, combine ground turkey, breadcrumbs, grated Parmesan cheese, egg, minced garlic, chopped fresh parsley, dried oregano, salt, and pepper. Mix until well combined.
3. Shape the turkey mixture into meatballs, about 1 inch in diameter.
4. Heat olive oil in a skillet over medium-high heat. Add the meatballs to the skillet and cook until browned on all sides, about 2-3 minutes per side.
5. Transfer the browned meatballs to a baking sheet lined with parchment paper.
6. Bake the meatballs in the preheated oven for 10-12 minutes, or until cooked through and no longer pink in the center.

Nutritional Information (per serving):

- Carbs: 5g
- Sodium: 70mg
- Potassium: 230mg
- Phosphorus: 120mg
- Protein: 25g

Baked Chicken Parmesan

Prep Time: 10 minutes | **Cook Time:** 20 minutes | **Servings:** 4

Ingredients:

- 4 boneless, skinless chicken breasts
- 1/2 cup breadcrumbs
- 1/4 cup grated Parmesan cheese
- 1 teaspoon dried basil
- 1 teaspoon dried oregano
- 1/2 teaspoon garlic powder
- Salt and pepper to taste
- Olive oil cooking spray
- 1 cup low-sodium marinara sauce
- 1/2 cup shredded mozzarella cheese
- Chopped fresh parsley, for garnish (optional)

Instructions:

1. Preheat your oven to 400°F (200°C).
2. In a shallow dish, combine breadcrumbs, grated Parmesan cheese, dried basil, dried oregano, garlic powder, salt, and pepper.
3. Dredge each chicken breast in the breadcrumb mixture, ensuring they are evenly coated.
4. Place the coated chicken breasts on a baking sheet lined with parchment paper.
5. Spray the tops of the chicken breasts with olive oil cooking spray.
6. Bake the chicken in the preheated oven for 15-20 minutes, or until the chicken is cooked through and reaches an internal temperature of 165°F (74°C).
7. Take out the chicken from the oven and top each breast with low-sodium marinara sauce and shredded mozzarella cheese.
8. Return the chicken to the oven and bake for an additional 5-7 minutes, or until the cheese is melted and bubbly.
9. Garnish with chopped fresh parsley before serving, if desired.

Nutritional Information (per serving):

- Carbs: 7g
- Sodium: 220mg
- Potassium: 280mg
- Phosphorus: 230mg
- Protein: 32g

Lemon Garlic Tilapia

Prep Time: 10 minutes | **Cook Time:** 15 minutes | **Servings:** 4

Ingredients:

- 4 tilapia fillets
- 2 tablespoons olive oil
- 2 cloves garlic, minced
- Zest of 1 lemon
- Juice of 1 lemon
- 1 tablespoon chopped fresh parsley
- Salt and pepper to taste

Instructions:

1. Preheat your oven to 400°F (200°C).
2. Place the tilapia fillets on a baking sheet lined with parchment paper.
3. In a small bowl, mix together the olive oil, minced garlic, lemon zest, lemon juice, chopped fresh parsley, salt, and pepper.
4. Brush the mixture over the tilapia fillets, ensuring they are evenly coated.
5. Bake the tilapia in the preheated oven for 12-15 minutes, or until the fish is opaque and flakes easily with a fork.
6. Once baked, take out the tilapia from the oven and let it rest for a few minutes before serving.

Nutritional Information (per serving):

- Carbs: 0g
- Sodium: 70mg
- Potassium: 200mg
- Phosphorus: 120mg
- Protein: 22g

Beef and Broccoli

Prep Time: 10 minutes | **Cook Time:** 15 minutes | **Servings:** 4

Ingredients:

- 1 pound beef sirloin steak, thinly sliced
- 2 tablespoons low-sodium soy sauce
- 2 cloves garlic, minced
- 1 tablespoon grated fresh ginger
- 2 cups broccoli florets
- 1 tablespoon olive oil
- 1/2 cup low-sodium beef broth
- 1 tablespoon cornstarch
- Salt and pepper to taste

Instructions:

1. In a bowl, marinate the thinly sliced beef sirloin steak with low-sodium soy sauce, minced garlic, and grated fresh ginger. Set aside for 10 minutes.
2. Heat olive oil in a large skillet or wok over medium-high heat.
3. Add the marinated beef slices to the skillet. Stir-fry for about 2-3 minutes, or until browned on all sides.
4. Add broccoli florets to the skillet and stir-fry for another 2-3 minutes, or until they are tender-crisp.
5. In a small bowl, mix together low-sodium beef broth and cornstarch to make a slurry.
6. Pour the slurry into the skillet and stir adequately to combine. Cook for an additional 1-2 minutes, or until the sauce thickens.
7. Season with salt and pepper to taste.
8. Serve the beef and broccoli hot over cooked rice or noodles.

Nutritional Information (per serving):

- Carbs: 5g
- Sodium: 150mg
- Potassium: 300mg
- Phosphorus: 200mg
- Protein: 25g

Mushroom Risotto

Prep Time: 10 minutes | **Cook Time:** 20 minutes | **Servings:** 4

Ingredients:

- 1 tablespoon olive oil
- 1 onion, finely chopped
- 2 cloves garlic, minced
- 1 cup Arborio rice
- 1/2 cup dry white wine
- 2 cups low-sodium vegetable broth
- 1 cup sliced mushrooms
- 1/4 cup grated Parmesan cheese
- Salt and pepper to taste
- Chopped fresh parsley for garnish (optional)

Instructions:

1. In a large skillet, heat olive oil over medium heat.
2. Add finely chopped onion and minced garlic to the skillet. Sauté until onion is translucent.
3. Add Arborio rice to the skillet and cook for 1-2 minutes, stirring constantly, until the rice is well coated with oil.
4. Pour in dry white wine and cook until it is absorbed by the rice, stirring frequently.
5. Gradually add low-sodium vegetable broth to the skillet, about 1/2 cup at a time, stirring constantly and allowing the liquid to be absorbed before adding more.
6. Stir in sliced mushrooms during the last 5 minutes of cooking.
7. Once the rice is creamy and tender, stir in grated Parmesan cheese.
8. Season with salt and pepper to taste.
9. Garnish with chopped fresh parsley before serving, if desired.

Nutritional Information (per serving):

- Carbs: 38g
- Sodium: 150mg
- Potassium: 200mg
- Phosphorus: 100mg
- Protein: 6g

Spinach and Feta Stuffed Chicken

Prep Time: 10 minutes | **Cook Time:** 20 minutes | **Servings:** 4

Ingredients:

- 4 boneless, skinless chicken breasts
- 2 cups fresh spinach leaves
- 1/2 cup crumbled feta cheese
- 2 cloves garlic, minced
- 1 tablespoon olive oil
- Salt and pepper to taste
- Toothpicks

Instructions:

1. Preheat your oven to 375°F (190°C).
2. Using a sharp knife, carefully cut a pocket into each chicken breast, being careful not to cut all the way through.
3. In a skillet, heat olive oil over medium heat. Add minced garlic and cook for about 1 minute until fragrant.
4. Add fresh spinach leaves to the skillet and cook until wilted, about 2-3 minutes.
5. Take out the skillet from the heat and stir in crumbled feta cheese. Allow the mixture to cool slightly.
6. Stuff each chicken breast with the spinach and feta mixture, using toothpicks to secure the openings.
7. Season the stuffed chicken breasts with salt and pepper.
8. Place the stuffed chicken breasts in a baking dish and bake in the preheated oven for 18-20 minutes, or until the chicken is cooked through and no longer pink in the center.
9. Once baked, take out the toothpicks from the chicken before serving.

Nutritional Information (per serving):

- Carbs: 2g
- Sodium: 180mg
- Potassium: 280mg
- Phosphorus: 200mg
- Protein: 30g

Lentil Curry

Prep Time: 10 minutes | **Cook Time:** 20 minutes | **Servings:** 4

Ingredients:

- 1 cup dried lentils, rinsed
- 2 cups water
- 1 tablespoon olive oil
- 1 onion, diced
- 2 cloves garlic, minced
- 1 tablespoon grated fresh ginger
- 1 tablespoon curry powder
- 1/2 teaspoon ground cumin
- 1/2 teaspoon ground turmeric
- 1/4 teaspoon cayenne pepper (optional)
- 1 can (14.5 ounces) low-sodium diced tomatoes, undrained
- Salt and pepper to taste
- Chopped fresh cilantro for garnish (optional)

Instructions:

1. In a saucepan, combine dried lentils and water. Bring to a boil, then reduce heat to low, cover, and simmer for 15-20 minutes, or until lentils are tender.
2. In a separate skillet, heat olive oil over medium heat. Add diced onion and cook until translucent.
3. Add minced garlic, grated fresh ginger, curry powder, ground cumin, ground turmeric, and cayenne pepper (if using) to the skillet. Cook for about 1 minute until fragrant.
4. Add low-sodium diced tomatoes to the skillet, along with their juices. Stir adequately to combine.
5. Once the lentils are tender, add them to the skillet with the tomato mixture. Stir to combine.
6. Simmer the lentil curry for an additional 5-10 minutes, allowing the flavors to meld together.
7. Season with salt and pepper to taste.
8. Garnish with chopped fresh cilantro before serving, if desired.

Nutritional Information (per serving):

- Carbs: 30g
- Sodium: 50mg
- Potassium: 400mg
- Phosphorus: 150mg
- Protein: 15g

Snacks

Apple Slices with Peanut Butter

Prep Time: 10 minutes | **Cook Time:** 0 minutes | **Servings:** 2

Ingredients:

- 1 medium apple, sliced
- 2 tablespoons peanut butter, unsalted
- 1 tablespoon honey
- 1 tablespoon chopped almonds, unsalted

Instructions:

1. Prepare ingredients: Wash and slice the apple. Chop the almonds.
2. Spread Peanut Butter: Spread 1 tablespoon of unsalted peanut butter evenly onto each apple slice.
3. Drizzle with Honey: Drizzle ½ tablespoon of honey over each apple slice topped with peanut butter.
4. Garnish with Almonds: Sprinkle chopped unsalted almonds over the apple slices.
5. Serve: Arrange the apple slices on a plate and serve immediately.

Nutritional Information (per serving):

- Carbs: 21g
- Sodium: 2mg
- Potassium: 140mg
- Phosphorus: 40mg
- Protein: 4g

Trail Mix

Prep Time: 10 minutes | **Cook Time:** 0 minutes | **Servings:** 4

Ingredients:

- ½ cup unsalted almonds
- ½ cup unsalted cashews
- ½ cup unsalted pumpkin seeds
- ½ cup dried cranberries
- ¼ cup unsalted sunflower seeds

Instructions:

1. Prepare ingredients: If needed, chop the almonds and cashews.
2. Combine **Ingredients:** In a mixing bowl, put in the almonds, cashews, pumpkin seeds, dried cranberries, and sunflower seeds.
3. Mix adequately: Mix all the ingredients until evenly distributed.
4. Portion: Divide the trail mix into 4 equal portions.
5. Serve or Store: Serve immediately or store in an airtight container for later consumption.

Nutritional Information (per serving):

- Carbs: 18g
- Sodium: 3mg
- Potassium: 150mg
- Phosphorus: 75mg
- Protein: 7g

Greek Yogurt

Prep Time: 5 minutes | **Cook Time:** 0 minutes | **Servings:** 2

Ingredients:

- 1 cup low-fat Greek yogurt
- ½ cup sliced strawberries
- ¼ cup blueberries
- 1 tablespoon honey
- 1 tablespoon chopped walnuts

Instructions:

1. Slice the strawberries and chop the walnuts if necessary.
2. In two serving bowls, divide the low-fat Greek yogurt equally.
3. Add ¼ cup of sliced strawberries and ⅛ cup of blueberries to each bowl.
4. Drizzle ½ tablespoon of honey over each serving of yogurt and fruit.
5. Sprinkle ½ tablespoon of chopped walnuts over each serving.
6. Serve immediately.

Nutritional Information (per serving):

- Carbs: 18g
- Sodium: 35mg
- Potassium: 180mg
- Phosphorus: 90mg
- Protein: 12g

Cheese and Crackers

Prep Time: 10 minutes | **Cook Time:** 0 minutes | **Servings:** 4

Ingredients:

- 4 ounces low-sodium cheese slices
- 16 whole wheat crackers
- ½ cup cherry tomatoes, halved
- ½ cup cucumber, sliced
- Fresh parsley for garnish

Instructions:

1. Prepare ingredients: Halve the cherry tomatoes, slice the cucumber, and set aside.
2. Assemble: On a serving platter, arrange the low-sodium cheese slices and whole wheat crackers.
3. Add Tomatoes and Cucumber: Place the halved cherry tomatoes and sliced cucumber on the platter alongside the cheese and crackers.
4. Garnish with Parsley: Sprinkle fresh parsley over the cheese and crackers for garnish.
5. Serve: Serve immediately as a kidney-friendly snack option.

Nutritional Information (per serving):

- Carbs: 16g
- Sodium: 120mg
- Potassium: 100mg
- Phosphorus: 80mg
- Protein: 8g

Rice Cakes with Hummus

Prep Time: 10 minutes | **Cook Time:** 0 minutes | **Servings:** 2

Ingredients:

- 4 rice cakes
- ½ cup low-sodium hummus
- ½ cup cucumber, sliced
- ½ cup carrot, sliced
- 2 tablespoons chopped fresh parsley

Instructions:

1. Prepare ingredients: Slice the cucumber and carrot, and chop the fresh parsley.
2. Spread Hummus: Spread 2 tablespoons of low-sodium hummus evenly onto each rice cake.
3. Add Cucumber and Carrot: Place the sliced cucumber and carrot on top of the hummus-covered rice cakes.
4. Garnish with Parsley: Sprinkle chopped fresh parsley over the rice cakes.
5. Serve: Serve immediately as a kidney-friendly snack option.

Nutritional Information (per serving):

- Carbs: 23g
- Sodium: 120mg
- Potassium: 140mg
- Phosphorus: 80mg
- Protein: 7g

Mixed Nuts

Prep Time: 5 minutes | **Cook Time:** 10 minutes | **Servings:** 4

Ingredients:

- 1 cup unsalted almonds
- 1 cup unsalted cashews
- ½ cup unsalted walnuts
- ½ cup unsalted peanuts
- ½ teaspoon olive oil
- ½ teaspoon garlic powder
- ½ teaspoon onion powder
- ½ teaspoon paprika
- ¼ teaspoon black pepper

Instructions:

1. Prepare ingredients: Preheat oven to 350°F (175°C). Measure out the unsalted almonds, cashews, walnuts, and peanuts.
2. Mix Nuts: In a mixing bowl, combine all the unsalted almonds, cashews, walnuts, and peanuts.
3. Season Nuts: Drizzle olive oil over the mixed nuts. Add garlic powder, onion powder, paprika, and black pepper. Toss until the nuts are evenly coated with the seasoning.
4. Roast Nuts: Spread the seasoned nuts evenly on a baking sheet. Roast in the preheated oven for 8-10 minutes, or until lightly golden and fragrant. Keep an eye on them to prevent burning.
5. Cool: Allow the nuts to cool completely before serving or storing.
6. Serve or Store: Serve as a snack or store in an airtight container for later consumption.

Nutritional Information (per serving):

- Carbs: 10g
- Sodium: 2mg
- Potassium: 120mg
- Phosphorus: 80mg
- Protein: 7g

Carrot Sticks with Hummus

Prep Time: 10 minutes | **Cook Time:** 0 minutes | **Servings:** 4

Ingredients:

- 4 medium carrots, peeled and cut into sticks
- 1 cup low-sodium hummus
- 1 tablespoon chopped fresh parsley

Instructions:

1. Prepare ingredients: Peel the carrots and cut them into sticks. Chop the fresh parsley.
2. Serve with Hummus: Arrange the carrot sticks on a serving platter or individual plates.
3. Garnish with Parsley: Sprinkle chopped fresh parsley over the carrot sticks.
4. Serve: Serve alongside low-sodium hummus for dipping.

Nutritional Information (per serving):

- Carbs: 14g
- Sodium: 70mg
- Potassium: 250mg
- Phosphorus: 40mg
- Protein: 7g

Cottage Cheese

Prep Time: 5 minutes | **Cook Time:** 0 minutes | **Servings:** 2

Ingredients:

- 1 cup low-sodium cottage cheese
- ½ cup diced cucumber
- ½ cup diced tomatoes
- 1 tablespoon chopped fresh chives
- Black pepper to taste

Instructions:

1. Prepare ingredients: Dice the cucumber and tomatoes. Chop the fresh chives.
2. Combine **Ingredients:** In a mixing bowl, put in the low-sodium cottage cheese, diced cucumber, diced tomatoes, and chopped fresh chives.
3. Season: Add black pepper to taste and mix adequately to combine all the ingredients.
4. Serve: Divide the cottage cheese mixture into two servings and serve immediately.

Nutritional Information (per serving):

- Carbs: 8g
- Sodium: 150mg
- Potassium: 200mg
- Phosphorus: 120mg
- Protein: 15g

Popcorn

Prep Time: 5 minutes | **Cook Time:** 5 minutes | **Servings:** 4

Ingredients:

- ½ cup popcorn kernels
- 1 tablespoon olive oil
- Salt to taste

Instructions:

1. Prepare Pot: Place a large pot with a lid on the stove over medium heat.
2. Add Oil: Add the olive oil to the pot and allow it to heat up.
3. Add Kernels: Add the popcorn kernels to the pot and cover it with the lid.
4. Pop: Shake the pot occasionally to ensure even heating. Once the popping slows down, take out the pot from the heat.
5. Season: Sprinkle salt over the freshly popped popcorn according to your taste preference. Toss to distribute the salt evenly.
6. Serve: Serve immediately as a kidney-friendly snack option.

Nutritional Information (per serving):

- Carbs: 6g
- Sodium: 0mg
- Potassium: 60mg
- Phosphorus: 90mg
- Protein: 2g

Sliced Cucumber with Lemon

Prep Time: 5 minutes | **Cook Time:** 0 minutes | **Servings:** 2

Ingredients:

- 1 medium cucumber, thinly sliced
- 1 tablespoon fresh lemon juice
- 1 teaspoon lemon zest
- 1 tablespoon chopped fresh parsley
- Salt to taste

Instructions:

1. Prepare ingredients: Thinly slice the cucumber and chop the fresh parsley.
2. Combine: In a mixing bowl, put in the thinly sliced cucumber, fresh lemon juice, lemon zest, and chopped fresh parsley.
3. Season: Sprinkle salt to taste over the cucumber mixture and toss gently to combine.
4. Serve: Serve immediately as a kidney-friendly snack option.

Nutritional Information (per serving):

- Carbs: 5g
- Sodium: 5mg
- Potassium: 150mg
- Phosphorus: 20mg
- Protein: 1g

Fruit Salad

Prep Time: 10 minutes | **Cook Time:** 0 minutes | **Servings:** 4

Ingredients:

- 1 cup diced strawberries
- 1 cup diced pineapple
- 1 cup diced peaches
- 1 cup diced kiwi
- 1 tablespoon fresh lime juice
- 1 tablespoon honey
- 1 tablespoon chopped fresh mint leaves

Instructions:

1. Prepare ingredients: Dice the strawberries, pineapple, peaches, and kiwi.
2. Combine Fruits: In a large mixing bowl, put in the diced strawberries, pineapple, peaches, and kiwi.
3. Dress Salad: Drizzle fresh lime juice and honey over the fruit mixture.
4. Add Mint: Sprinkle chopped fresh mint leaves over the fruit salad.
5. Toss: Gently toss the fruit salad until all the ingredients are well combined and evenly coated with the lime juice, honey, and mint.
6. Serve: Serve immediately as a kidney-friendly dessert or snack option.

Nutritional Information (per serving):

- Carbs: 30g
- Sodium: 5mg
- Potassium: 300mg
- Phosphorus: 40mg
- Protein: 1g

Edamame

Prep Time: 5 minutes | **Cook Time:** 5 minutes | **Servings:** 4

Ingredients:

- 2 cups frozen shelled edamame
- Water for boiling
- Salt to taste

Instructions:

1. Boil Edamame: Bring a pot of water to a boil over high heat.
2. Add Edamame: Once the water is boiling, add the frozen shelled edamame to the pot.
3. Cook: Boil the edamame for 4-5 minutes, or until they are tender.
4. Drain: Drain the cooked edamame in a colander.
5. Season: Sprinkle salt to taste over the drained edamame and toss to coat evenly.
6. Serve: Serve immediately as a kidney-friendly snack option.

Nutritional Information (per serving):

- Carbs: 8g
- Sodium: 5mg
- Potassium: 130mg
- Phosphorus: 60mg
- Protein: 9g

Pretzels

Prep Time: 10 minutes | **Cook Time:** 15 minutes | **Servings:** 4

Ingredients:

- 2 cups all-purpose flour
- 1 tablespoon active dry yeast
- 1 teaspoon sugar
- ½ teaspoon salt
- ¾ cup warm water
- 1 egg, beaten
- Coarse salt for topping (optional)

Instructions:

1. Activate Yeast: In a small bowl, dissolve the sugar in warm water. Sprinkle the active dry yeast over the water and let it sit for 5 minutes until foamy.
2. Mix Dough: In a large mixing bowl, put in the all-purpose flour and salt. Pour in the activated yeast mixture and stir until a dough forms.
3. Knead Dough: Transfer the dough to a lightly floured surface and knead for 5-7 minutes, until the dough is smooth and elastic.
4. Shape Pretzels: Divide the dough into 8 equal portions. Roll each portion into a long rope, then shape into pretzels.
5. Boil Pretzels: Preheat the oven to 425°F (220°C). Bring a large pot of water to a boil. Carefully add the pretzels to the boiling water, one or two at a time, and boil for 30 seconds. Remove with a slotted spoon and place on a baking sheet lined with parchment paper.
6. Brush with Egg Wash: Brush the tops of the pretzels with beaten egg. Sprinkle coarse salt on top if desired.
7. Bake: Bake the pretzels in the preheated oven for 12-15 minutes, or until golden brown.
8. Cool and Serve: Allow the pretzels to cool slightly before serving. Enjoy them warm as a kidney-friendly snack option.

Nutritional Information (per serving):

- Carbs: 38g
- Sodium: 240mg
- Potassium: 50mg
- Phosphorus: 70mg
- Protein: 9g

Roasted Chickpeas

Prep Time: 5 minutes | **Cook Time:** 25 minutes | **Servings:** 4

Ingredients:

- 2 cans (15 ounces each) low-sodium chickpeas, drained and rinsed
- 1 tablespoon olive oil
- ½ teaspoon garlic powder
- ½ teaspoon onion powder
- ½ teaspoon paprika
- ¼ teaspoon black pepper

Instructions:

1. Preheat Oven: Preheat the oven to 400°F (200°C).
2. Dry Chickpeas: Pat the drained and rinsed chickpeas dry with paper towels or a clean kitchen towel. Remove any loose skins.
3. Season Chickpeas: In a mixing bowl, put in the dried chickpeas with olive oil, garlic powder, onion powder, paprika, and black pepper. Toss until the chickpeas are evenly coated with the seasoning.
4. Roast Chickpeas: Spread the seasoned chickpeas in a single layer on a baking sheet lined with parchment paper.
5. Bake: Roast the chickpeas in the preheated oven for 20-25 minutes, or until crispy and golden brown, shaking the pan halfway through cooking.
6. Cool and Serve: Allow the roasted chickpeas to cool slightly before serving. Enjoy them warm or at room temperature as a kidney-friendly snack option.

Nutritional Information (per serving):

- Carbs: 22g
- Sodium: 15mg
- Potassium: 190mg
- Phosphorus: 60mg
- Protein: 7g

Yogurt Bark

Prep Time: 10 minutes | **Cook Time:** 0 minutes | **Servings:** 6

Ingredients:

- 2 cups low-fat Greek yogurt
- 1 tablespoon honey
- ½ cup diced strawberries
- ½ cup blueberries
- 2 tablespoons chopped almonds, unsalted

Instructions:

1. Prepare ingredients: Dice the strawberries and chop the almonds if necessary.
2. Mix Yogurt: In a mixing bowl, put in the low-fat Greek yogurt and honey until well mixed.
3. Spread Yogurt: Line a baking sheet with parchment paper. Spread the yogurt mixture evenly onto the parchment paper, creating a rectangular shape about ¼ inch thick.
4. Add Fruit and Nuts: Sprinkle the diced strawberries, blueberries, and chopped unsalted almonds over the yogurt mixture.
5. Freeze: Place the baking sheet in the freezer for at least 2 hours, or until the yogurt bark is firm.
6. Break into Pieces: Once frozen, take out the yogurt bark from the freezer and break it into pieces using your hands or a knife.
7. Serve: Serve immediately as a kidney-friendly dessert or snack option.

Nutritional Information (per serving):

- Carbs: 12g
- Sodium: 25mg
- Potassium: 110mg
- Phosphorus: 50mg
- Protein: 6g

Peanut Butter Banana Bites

Prep Time: 10 minutes | **Cook Time:** 0 minutes | **Servings:** 4

Ingredients:

- 2 large bananas
- ¼ cup peanut butter (unsalted)
- 2 tablespoons chopped almonds (unsalted)

Instructions:

1. Prepare ingredients: Peel the bananas and slice them into rounds, about ½ inch thick.
2. Assemble: Take half of the banana slices and spread about ½ teaspoon of peanut butter on each slice. Top each peanut butter-covered banana slice with another banana slice to create banana sandwiches.
3. Top with Almonds: Press a few chopped unsalted almonds onto the sides of each peanut butter-filled banana sandwich.
4. Serve: Serve immediately as a kidney-friendly snack option.

Nutritional Information (per serving):

- Carbs: 17g
- Sodium: 2mg
- Potassium: 230mg
- Phosphorus: 55mg
- Protein: 4g

Veggie Chips

Prep Time: 10 minutes | **Cook Time:** 20 minutes | **Servings:** 4

Ingredients:

- 2 large carrots
- 2 medium zucchinis
- 1 tablespoon olive oil
- Salt to taste

Instructions:

1. Preheat Oven: Preheat the oven to 375°F (190°C) and line a baking sheet with parchment paper.
2. Prepare Vegetables: Wash the carrots and zucchinis. Using a mandoline slicer or a sharp knife, slice the carrots and zucchinis into thin rounds.
3. Pat Dry: Pat the sliced carrots and zucchinis dry with a clean kitchen towel to remove excess moisture.
4. Toss with Oil: In a mixing bowl, toss the sliced carrots and zucchinis with olive oil until they are evenly coated.
5. Arrange on Baking Sheet: Spread the coated vegetable slices in a single layer on the prepared baking sheet.
6. Bake: Bake in the preheated oven for 15-20 minutes, or until the vegetable chips are golden and crispy, flipping halfway through cooking.
7. Season: Sprinkle salt to taste over the hot veggie chips immediately after removing them from the oven.
8. Cool and Serve: Allow the veggie chips to cool slightly before serving. Enjoy them warm or at room temperature as a kidney-friendly snack option.

Nutritional Information (per serving):

- Carbs: 8g
- Sodium: 60mg
- Potassium: 250mg
- Phosphorus: 40mg
- Protein: 1g

Desserts

Berry Crisp

Prep Time: 10 minutes | **Cook Time:** 20 minutes | **Servings:** 4

Ingredients:

- 2 cups mixed berries (fresh or frozen)
- 1/4 cup granulated sugar
- 1/2 cup oats
- 1/4 cup all-purpose flour
- 1/4 cup brown sugar
- 1/4 teaspoon cinnamon
- 1/4 cup unsalted butter, cold and diced

Instructions:

1. Preheat your oven to 375°F (190°C).
2. In a bowl, toss the mixed berries with the granulated sugar until evenly coated, then transfer them to a baking dish.
3. In another bowl, put in the oats, all-purpose flour, brown sugar, and cinnamon. Mix adequately.
4. Add the diced unsalted butter to the oat mixture. Using your fingers or a fork, mix until the mixture resembles coarse crumbs.
5. Sprinkle the oat mixture evenly over the berries in the baking dish.
6. Bake in the preheated oven for about 20 minutes, or until the topping is golden brown and the berries are bubbling.
7. Remove from the oven and let it cool slightly before serving.
8. Serve warm, optionally with a scoop of vanilla ice cream or whipped cream.

Nutritional Information:

Carbs: 25g

Sodium: 2mg

Potassium: 103mg

Phosphorus: 64mg

Protein: 2g

Poached Pears

Prep Time: 10 minutes | **Cook Time:** 20 minutes | **Servings:** 4

Ingredients:

- 4 ripe pears, peeled and cored
- 2 cups water
- 1/2 cup granulated sugar
- 1 cinnamon stick
- 1 teaspoon vanilla extract
- 1/2 teaspoon lemon zest

Instructions:

1. In a pot, put in the water, granulated sugar, cinnamon stick, vanilla extract, and lemon zest. Bring the mixture to a simmer over medium heat, stirring occasionally until the sugar dissolves.
2. Once the sugar has dissolved, add the peeled and cored pears to the pot, ensuring they are fully submerged in the liquid.
3. Reduce the heat to low and let the pears simmer gently for about 15-20 minutes, or until they are tender when pierced with a fork.
4. Once the pears are tender, remove them from the poaching liquid and set them aside.
5. Increase the heat to medium-high and let the poaching liquid simmer for an additional 5-10 minutes, or until it has reduced and thickened slightly.
6. Take out the cinnamon stick from the poaching liquid and discard.
7. Serve the poached pears warm or chilled, drizzled with the reduced poaching liquid.

Nutritional Information:

- Carbs: 28g
- Sodium: 1mg
- Potassium: 177mg
- Phosphorus: 11mg
- Protein: 0.3g

Rice Pudding

Prep Time: 5 minutes | **Cook Time:** 25 minutes | **Servings:** 4

Ingredients:

- 1/2 cup white rice
- 2 cups low-fat milk
- 1/4 cup granulated sugar
- 1/2 teaspoon vanilla extract
- 1/4 teaspoon ground cinnamon
- 1/4 cup raisins (optional)

Instructions:

1. In a saucepan, put in the white rice and low-fat milk. Bring to a boil over medium-high heat, then reduce the heat to low and simmer, uncovered, stirring occasionally, for about 15-20 minutes, or until the rice is tender and the mixture has thickened.
2. Stir in the granulated sugar, vanilla extract, ground cinnamon, and raisins (if using). Continue to cook for an additional 5 minutes, stirring occasionally.
3. Take out the rice pudding from the heat and let it cool slightly before serving.
4. Serve the rice pudding warm or chilled, optionally sprinkled with an extra dash of cinnamon on top.

Nutritional Information:

- Carbs: 34g
- Sodium: 62mg
- Potassium: 147mg
- Phosphorus: 97mg
- Protein: 5g

Angel Food Cake

Prep Time: 10 minutes | **Cook Time:** 25 minutes | **Servings:** 8

Ingredients:

- 1 cup cake flour
- 1 1/2 cups granulated sugar, divided
- 12 large egg whites, at room temperature
- 1 teaspoon cream of tartar
- 1 teaspoon vanilla extract
- 1/4 teaspoon salt

Instructions:

1. Preheat your oven to 350°F (175°C).
2. In a bowl, sift together the cake flour and 1/2 cup of granulated sugar.
3. In a separate large bowl, beat the egg whites with an electric mixer until foamy.
4. Add the cream of tartar, vanilla extract, and salt to the egg whites. Continue to beat until soft peaks form.
5. Gradually add the remaining 1 cup of granulated sugar, about 2 tablespoons at a time, while continuing to beat the egg whites until stiff peaks form.
6. Gently fold the sifted flour mixture into the beaten egg whites, about 1/4 cup at a time, until fully incorporated.
7. Spoon the batter into an ungreased angel food cake pan, spreading it evenly.
8. Bake in the preheated oven for 25-30 minutes, or until the top of the cake is golden brown and springs back when lightly touched.
9. Take out the cake from the oven and immediately invert the pan onto a cooling rack, allowing the cake to cool completely while hanging upside down.
10. Once cooled, carefully run a knife around the edges of the pan to loosen the cake, then remove it from the pan.
11. Slice and serve the angel food cake plain or with fresh berries, if desired.

Nutritional Information:

- Carbs: 32g
- Sodium: 92mg
- Potassium: 86mg
- Phosphorus: 86mg
- Protein: 5g

Banana Ice Cream

Prep Time: 5 minutes | **Cook Time:** 0 minutes | **Servings:** 2

Ingredients:

- 2 ripe bananas, sliced and frozen
- 1/4 cup low-fat milk
- 1/2 teaspoon vanilla extract
- Optional toppings: chopped nuts, sliced fruit

Instructions:

1. Place the sliced and frozen bananas in a blender or food processor.
2. Add the low-fat milk and vanilla extract to the blender.
3. Blend the mixture until smooth and creamy, scraping down the sides of the blender as needed.
4. Once the mixture reaches a smooth consistency, transfer it to a freezer-safe container.
5. Freeze the banana mixture for about 20-30 minutes, or until it firms up slightly.
6. Take out the container from the freezer and scoop the banana ice cream into bowls.
7. Serve immediately, topped with your favorite optional toppings if desired.

Nutritional Information:

- Carbs: 26g
- Sodium: 9mg
- Potassium: 422mg
- Phosphorus: 32mg
- Protein: 2g

Strawberry Sorbet

Prep Time: 10 minutes | **Cook Time:** 0 minutes | **Servings:** 4

Ingredients:

- 4 cups frozen strawberries
- 1/4 cup water
- 1/4 cup granulated sugar
- 1 tablespoon lemon juice

Instructions:

1. In a blender or food processor, put in the frozen strawberries, water, granulated sugar, and lemon juice.
2. Blend the mixture until smooth, scraping down the sides of the blender or food processor as needed.
3. Once the mixture reaches a smooth consistency, transfer it to a shallow dish or container.
4. Place the dish or container in the freezer for about 20-30 minutes, or until the sorbet firms up slightly.
5. Take out the sorbet from the freezer and scoop it into bowls to serve.

Nutritional Information:

- Carbs: 24g
- Sodium: 1mg
- Potassium: 201mg
- Phosphorus: 34mg
- Protein: 1g

Chocolate Avocado Mousse

Prep Time: 10 minutes | **Cook Time:** 0 minutes | **Servings:** 4

Ingredients:

- 2 ripe avocados, peeled and pitted
- 1/4 cup unsweetened cocoa powder
- 1/4 cup low-fat milk
- 1/4 cup granulated sugar
- 1 teaspoon vanilla extract
- Pinch of salt
- Optional toppings: sliced strawberries, chopped nuts

Instructions:

1. In a blender or food processor, put in the peeled and pitted avocados, unsweetened cocoa powder, low-fat milk, granulated sugar, vanilla extract, and a pinch of salt.
2. Blend the mixture until smooth and creamy, scraping down the sides of the blender or food processor as needed.
3. Once the mixture reaches a smooth consistency, transfer it to serving bowls or glasses.
4. Refrigerate the mousse for about 20-30 minutes, or until it firms up slightly.
5. Take out the mousse from the refrigerator and garnish with optional toppings such as sliced strawberries or chopped nuts before serving.

Nutritional Information:

- Carbs: 17g
- Sodium: 36mg
- Potassium: 487mg
- Phosphorus: 124mg
- Protein: 3g

Lemon Poppy Seed Muffins

Prep Time: 10 minutes | **Cook Time:** 20 minutes | **Servings:** 12

Ingredients:

- 2 cups all-purpose flour
- 1/2 cup granulated sugar
- 2 teaspoons baking powder
- 1/2 teaspoon baking soda
- Pinch of salt
- Zest of 2 lemons
- 1/4 cup lemon juice
- 1/2 cup low-fat milk
- 1/4 cup unsalted butter, melted
- 2 large eggs
- 1 tablespoon poppy seeds

Instructions:

1. Preheat your oven to 375°F (190°C). Line a muffin tin with paper liners or grease it lightly.
2. In a large mixing bowl, put in the all-purpose flour, granulated sugar, baking powder, baking soda, pinch of salt, and lemon zest.
3. In a separate bowl, whisk together the lemon juice, low-fat milk, melted unsalted butter, and eggs until well combined.
4. Pour the wet ingredients into the dry ingredients and mix until just combined. Do not overmix.
5. Gently fold in the poppy seeds until evenly distributed throughout the batter.
6. Divide the batter evenly among the prepared muffin cups, filling each about two-thirds full.
7. Bake in the preheated oven for 18-20 minutes, or until the muffins are golden brown and a toothpick inserted into the center comes out clean.
8. Take out the muffins from the oven and let them cool in the tin for a few minutes before transferring them to a wire rack to cool completely.

Nutritional Information:

- Carbs: 26g
- Sodium: 105mg
- Potassium: 66mg
- Phosphorus: 76mg
- Protein: 3g

Pumpkin Pie

Prep Time: 10 minutes | **Cook Time:** 25 minutes | **Servings:** 8

Ingredients:

- 1 (15-ounce) can pumpkin puree
- 1/2 cup low-fat milk
- 1/2 cup granulated sugar
- 2 large eggs
- 1 teaspoon ground cinnamon
- 1/2 teaspoon ground ginger
- 1/4 teaspoon ground nutmeg
- 1/4 teaspoon ground cloves
- 1/4 teaspoon salt
- 1 (9-inch) pre-made pie crust (store-bought or homemade)

Instructions:

1. Preheat your oven to 425°F (220°C).
2. In a large mixing bowl, put in the pumpkin puree, low-fat milk, granulated sugar, eggs, ground cinnamon, ground ginger, ground nutmeg, ground cloves, and salt. Mix until well combined.
3. Pour the pumpkin mixture into the pre-made pie crust, spreading it evenly.
4. Bake the pie in the preheated oven for 15 minutes.
5. After 15 minutes, reduce the oven temperature to 350°F (175°C) and continue to bake for an additional 10 minutes, or until the filling is set.
6. Take out the pie from the oven and let it cool completely before serving.

Nutritional Information:

- Carbs: 24g
- Sodium: 161mg
- Potassium: 201mg
- Phosphorus: 67mg
- Protein: 3g

Oatmeal Raisin Cookies

Prep Time: 10 minutes | **Cook Time:** 15 minutes | **Servings:** 24

Ingredients:

- 1 cup old-fashioned oats
- 3/4 cup all-purpose flour
- 1/2 teaspoon baking soda
- 1/2 teaspoon ground cinnamon
- 1/4 teaspoon salt
- 1/2 cup unsalted butter, softened
- 1/2 cup granulated sugar
- 1/4 cup brown sugar
- 1 large egg
- 1 teaspoon vanilla extract
- 1/2 cup raisins

Instructions:

1. Preheat your oven to 350°F (175°C). Line a baking sheet with parchment paper or lightly grease it.
2. In a bowl, put in the old-fashioned oats, all-purpose flour, baking soda, ground cinnamon, and salt.
3. In a separate large mixing bowl, cream together the softened unsalted butter, granulated sugar, and brown sugar until smooth.
4. Beat in the egg and vanilla extract until well combined.
5. Gradually add the dry ingredients to the wet ingredients, mixing until a dough forms.
6. Fold in the raisins until evenly distributed throughout the dough.
7. Drop tablespoon-sized portions of dough onto the prepared baking sheet, spacing them about 2 inches apart.
8. Flatten each cookie slightly with the back of a spoon or your hand.
9. Bake in the preheated oven for 10-12 minutes, or until the edges are golden brown.
10. Take out the cookies from the oven and let them cool on the baking sheet for a few minutes before transferring them to a wire rack to cool completely.

Nutritional Information:

- Carbs: 13g
- Sodium: 51mg
- Potassium: 59mg
- Phosphorus: 39mg
- Protein: 1g

Peach Cobbler

Prep Time: 10 minutes | **Cook Time:** 25 minutes | **Servings:** 6

Ingredients:

- 4 cups sliced fresh peaches (or thawed frozen peaches)
- 1/4 cup granulated sugar
- 1 tablespoon lemon juice
- 1/2 teaspoon ground cinnamon
- 1 cup all-purpose flour
- 1/4 cup granulated sugar
- 1 teaspoon baking powder
- Pinch of salt
- 1/2 cup low-fat milk
- 1/4 cup unsalted butter, melted

Instructions:

1. Preheat your oven to 375°F (190°C).
2. In a mixing bowl, put in the sliced fresh peaches (or thawed frozen peaches) with the granulated sugar, lemon juice, and ground cinnamon. Stir until the peaches are evenly coated, then transfer them to a baking dish.
3. In another bowl, whisk together the all-purpose flour, granulated sugar, baking powder, and pinch of salt.
4. Gradually stir in the low-fat milk until a smooth batter forms.
5. Pour the melted unsalted butter into the batter and mix until well combined.
6. Spoon the batter evenly over the peaches in the baking dish.
7. Bake in the preheated oven for 25-30 minutes, or until the cobbler topping is golden brown and cooked through.
8. Take out the cobbler from the oven and let it cool slightly before serving.

Nutritional Information:

- Carbs: 37g
- Sodium: 52mg
- Potassium: 223mg
- Phosphorus: 72mg
- Protein: 3g

Apple Cinnamon Bars

Prep Time: 10 minutes | **Cook Time:** 20 minutes | **Servings:** 12

Ingredients:

- 1 1/2 cups all-purpose flour
- 1 cup old-fashioned oats
- 1/2 cup brown sugar
- 1 teaspoon ground cinnamon
- 1/2 teaspoon baking powder
- 1/4 teaspoon salt
- 1/2 cup unsalted butter, melted
- 2 cups diced apples (such as Granny Smith)
- 1 tablespoon lemon juice
- 1 tablespoon granulated sugar

Instructions:

1. Preheat your oven to 350°F (175°C). Grease or line a 9x9-inch baking pan with parchment paper.
2. In a large mixing bowl, put in the all-purpose flour, old-fashioned oats, brown sugar, ground cinnamon, baking powder, and salt.
3. Pour the melted unsalted butter over the dry ingredients and mix until crumbly.
4. Press two-thirds of the mixture evenly into the bottom of the prepared baking pan to form the crust.
5. In another bowl, toss the diced apples with lemon juice and granulated sugar until well coated.
6. Spread the apple mixture evenly over the crust in the baking pan.
7. Sprinkle the remaining oat mixture evenly over the top of the apples.
8. Bake in the preheated oven for 20-25 minutes, or until the top is golden brown and the apples are tender.
9. Remove from the oven and let cool completely before cutting into bars.

Nutritional Information:

- Carbs: 29g
- Sodium: 50mg
- Potassium: 88mg
- Phosphorus: 59mg
- Protein: 2g

Coconut Macaroons

Prep Time: 10 minutes | **Cook Time:** 15 minutes | **Servings:** 12

Ingredients:

- 3 cups unsweetened shredded coconut
- 1/2 cup granulated sugar
- 2 large egg whites
- 1/2 teaspoon vanilla extract
- Pinch of salt

Instructions:

1. Preheat your oven to 350°F (175°C). Line a baking sheet with parchment paper.
2. In a mixing bowl, put in the unsweetened shredded coconut, granulated sugar, egg whites, vanilla extract, and a pinch of salt. Mix until well combined.
3. Using a spoon or cookie scoop, scoop out portions of the coconut mixture and shape them into balls using your hands. Place the balls onto the prepared baking sheet, spacing them about 1 inch apart.
4. Bake in the preheated oven for 12-15 minutes, or until the macaroons are golden brown around the edges.
5. Remove from the oven and let the macaroons cool on the baking sheet for a few minutes before transferring them to a wire rack to cool completely.

Nutritional Information:

- Carbs: 8g
- Sodium: 12mg
- Potassium: 64mg
- Phosphorus: 45mg
- Protein: 1g

Berry Smoothie Bowl

Prep Time: 10 minutes | **Cook Time:** 0 minutes | **Servings:** 2

Ingredients:

- 1 cup frozen mixed berries
- 1 ripe banana, sliced
- 1/2 cup low-fat yogurt
- 1/4 cup low-fat milk
- 2 tablespoons rolled oats
- 1 tablespoon honey
- Optional toppings: sliced almonds, shredded coconut, fresh berries

Instructions:

1. In a blender, put in the frozen mixed berries, sliced ripe banana, low-fat yogurt, low-fat milk, rolled oats, and honey.
2. Blend the mixture until smooth and creamy, adding more milk if needed to reach your desired consistency.
3. Pour the smoothie into bowls.
4. Top the smoothie bowls with optional toppings such as sliced almonds, shredded coconut, and fresh berries.
5. Serve immediately and enjoy!

Nutritional Information:

- Carbs: 28g
- Sodium: 38mg
- Potassium: 322mg
- Phosphorus: 127mg
- Protein: 5g

Greek Yogurt Cheesecake

Prep Time: 10 minutes | **Cook Time:** 25 minutes | **Servings:** 8

Ingredients:

- 1 cup low-fat Greek yogurt
- 8 ounces low-fat cream cheese, softened
- 1/2 cup granulated sugar
- 2 large eggs
- 1 teaspoon vanilla extract
- 1/4 cup all-purpose flour
- 1/4 teaspoon salt

Instructions:

1. Preheat your oven to 325°F (160°C). Grease a 9-inch pie dish or springform pan.
2. In a large mixing bowl, put in the low-fat Greek yogurt, softened low-fat cream cheese, and granulated sugar. Mix until smooth and creamy.
3. Add the eggs, one at a time, mixing well after each addition.
4. Stir in the vanilla extract.
5. Gradually add the all-purpose flour and salt, mixing until fully incorporated and the batter is smooth.
6. Pour the batter into the prepared pie dish or springform pan.
7. Bake in the preheated oven for 25-30 minutes, or until the edges are set and the center is slightly jiggly.
8. Remove from the oven and let the cheesecake cool completely at room temperature.
9. Once cooled, refrigerate for at least 2 hours before serving.

Nutritional Information:

- Carbs: 16g
- Sodium: 196mg
- Potassium: 106mg
- Phosphorus: 83mg
- Protein: 7g

Chocolate Covered Strawberries

Prep Time: 10 minutes | **Cook Time:** 5 minutes | **Servings:** 12

Ingredients:

- 12 large strawberries
- 4 ounces dark chocolate (choose low-sodium, low-potassium, and low-phosphorus varieties if available)

Instructions:

1. Rinse the strawberries under cold water and pat them dry with paper towels.
2. Line a baking sheet with parchment paper.
3. In a microwave-safe bowl, break the dark chocolate into small pieces.
4. Microwave the chocolate in 30-second intervals, stirring between each interval, until fully melted and smooth.
5. Hold a strawberry by the stem and dip it into the melted chocolate, coating it halfway.
6. Allow any excess chocolate to drip off the strawberry, then place it on the prepared baking sheet.
7. Repeat the dipping process with the remaining strawberries.
8. Place the baking sheet in the refrigerator for about 10-15 minutes, or until the chocolate coating is set.
9. Once set, take out the chocolate-covered strawberries from the refrigerator and serve.

Nutritional Information:

- Carbs: 7g
- Sodium: 2mg
- Potassium: 61mg
- Phosphorus: 21mg
- Protein: 1g

Chia Seed Pudding

Prep Time: 5 minutes | **Cook Time:** 0 minutes | **Servings:** 2

Ingredients:

- 1/4 cup chia seeds
- 1 cup low-fat milk
- 1 tablespoon honey or maple syrup
- 1/2 teaspoon vanilla extract
- Optional toppings: sliced fruit, chopped nuts, shredded coconut

Instructions:

1. In a mixing bowl, put in the chia seeds, low-fat milk, honey or maple syrup, and vanilla extract. Stir adequately to combine.
2. Cover the bowl and refrigerate for at least 20-30 minutes, or until the mixture has thickened to a pudding-like consistency. Stir occasionally to prevent clumping.
3. Once the chia seed pudding has thickened, remove it from the refrigerator.
4. Divide the pudding into serving bowls.
5. Top with optional toppings such as sliced fruit, chopped nuts, or shredded coconut.
6. Serve chilled and enjoy!

Nutritional Information:

- Carbs: 15g
- Sodium: 48mg
- Potassium: 92mg
- Phosphorus: 115mg
- Protein: 5g

Beverages

Green Smoothie

Prep Time: 5 minutes | **Cook Time:** 0 minutes | **Servings:** 2

Ingredients:

- 2 cups fresh spinach leaves
- 1 ripe banana, peeled and sliced
- 1/2 cup chopped cucumber
- 1/2 cup chopped celery
- 1/2 cup unsweetened almond milk
- 1 tablespoon fresh lemon juice
- 1 tablespoon fresh parsley leaves
- 1/2 teaspoon grated ginger
- 1/2 cup ice cubes

Instructions:

1. In a blender, combine fresh spinach leaves, sliced banana, chopped cucumber, chopped celery, unsweetened almond milk, fresh lemon juice, parsley leaves, grated ginger, and ice cubes.
2. Blend until smooth and creamy.
3. Pour into glasses and serve immediately.

Nutritional Information (per serving):

- Carbs: 16g
- Sodium: 66mg
- Potassium: 400mg
- Phosphorus: 60mg
- Protein: 2g

Iced Herbal Tea

Prep Time: 5 minutes | **Cook Time:** 10 minutes | **Servings:** 4

Ingredients:

- 4 cups water
- 4 herbal tea bags (such as chamomile or mint)
- 1 tablespoon honey (optional)
- 1 lemon, sliced
- Ice cubes

Instructions:

1. Bring 4 cups of water to a boil in a pot.
2. Once boiling, remove from heat and add 4 herbal tea bags (such as chamomile or mint) to the water. Let steep for 5-10 minutes.
3. Take out the tea bags and discard.
4. Stir in 1 tablespoon of honey (optional) until dissolved.
5. Allow the tea to cool to room temperature.
6. Once cooled, transfer the tea to a pitcher and add sliced lemon.
7. Refrigerate until chilled.
8. Serve the tea over ice cubes.

Nutritional Information (per serving):

- Carbs: 5g
- Sodium: 2mg
- Potassium: 18mg
- Phosphorus: 4mg
- Protein: 0g

Fruit Infused Water

Prep Time: 5 minutes | **Cook Time:** 0 minutes | **Servings:** 4

Ingredients:

- 4 cups water
- 1 cup sliced strawberries
- 1/2 cup sliced cucumber
- 1/2 cup sliced lemon
- 1/4 cup fresh mint leaves
- Ice cubes

Instructions:

1. In a pitcher, combine 4 cups of water with 1 cup of sliced strawberries, 1/2 cup of sliced cucumber, 1/2 cup of sliced lemon, and 1/4 cup of fresh mint leaves.
2. Stir the ingredients gently to mix.
3. Refrigerate the infused water for at least 30 minutes to allow the flavors to meld.
4. Serve the infused water over ice cubes.

Nutritional Information (per serving):

- Carbs: 4g
- Sodium: 2mg
- Potassium: 55mg
- Phosphorus: 10mg
- Protein: 0g

Almond Milk

Prep Time: 10 minutes | **Cook Time:** 10 minutes | **Servings:** 4

Ingredients:

- 1 cup raw almonds
- 4 cups water
- Sweetener of choice (optional), such as stevia or erythritol

Instructions:

1. Place 1 cup of raw almonds in a bowl and cover with water. Allow them to soak for at least 4 hours or overnight.
2. Drain and rinse the soaked almonds.
3. In a blender, put in the soaked almonds with 4 cups of water.
4. Blend on high speed for 2-3 minutes until the almonds are finely ground and the mixture looks creamy.
5. Strain the almond mixture through a nut milk bag or cheesecloth into a clean container, squeezing to extract as much liquid as possible.
6. Sweeten the almond milk with your preferred sweetener, if desired, and stir until dissolved.
7. Transfer the almond milk to a sealed container and refrigerate. It will keep for about 3-4 days.

Nutritional Information (per serving):

- Carbs: 3g
- Sodium: 0mg
- Potassium: 65mg
- Phosphorus: 45mg
- Protein: 2g

Protein Shake

Prep Time: 5 minutes | **Cook Time:** 0 minutes | **Servings:** 1

Ingredients:

- 1 scoop low-phosphorus protein powder
- 1 cup unsweetened almond milk
- 1/2 banana, peeled and sliced
- 1 tablespoon almond butter
- 1/2 teaspoon cinnamon
- Ice cubes (optional)

Instructions:

1. In a blender, combine 1 scoop of low-phosphorus protein powder, 1 cup of unsweetened almond milk, 1/2 banana (peeled and sliced), 1 tablespoon of almond butter, and 1/2 teaspoon of cinnamon.
2. If desired, add ice cubes for a colder shake.
3. Blend on high speed until smooth and creamy.
4. Pour the protein shake into a glass and serve immediately.

Nutritional Information (per serving):

- Carbs: 18g
- Sodium: 120mg
- Potassium: 230mg
- Phosphorus: 150mg
- Protein: 20g

Vegetable Juice

Prep Time: 10 minutes | **Cook Time:** 0 minutes | **Servings:** 2

Ingredients:

- 2 large carrots, peeled and chopped
- 2 stalks celery, chopped
- 1 small beet, peeled and chopped
- 1/2 cucumber, chopped
- 1 handful spinach leaves
- 1/2 lemon, peeled
- 1-inch piece of ginger, peeled
- Water, as needed

Instructions:

1. In a juicer, add 2 large carrots (peeled and chopped), 2 stalks of celery (chopped), 1 small beet (peeled and chopped), 1/2 cucumber (chopped), 1 handful of spinach leaves, 1/2 lemon (peeled), and a 1-inch piece of ginger (peeled).
2. Turn on the juicer and process the vegetables and fruits until juiced.
3. If the juice is too thick, you can add a little water to thin it out to your desired consistency.
4. Once juiced, pour the vegetable juice into glasses and serve immediately.

Nutritional Information (per serving):

- Carbs: 15g
- Sodium: 110mg
- Potassium: 540mg
- Phosphorus: 80mg
- Protein: 3g

Coconut Water

Prep Time: 5 minutes | **Cook Time:** 0 minutes | **Servings:** 2

Ingredients:

- 1 fresh coconut
- Water

Instructions:

1. Using a cleaver or a heavy chef's knife, carefully crack open the coconut. Collect the coconut water in a clean container.
2. Strain the coconut water through a fine mesh sieve to remove any debris.
3. Optionally, you can transfer the coconut water to a blender and blend for a few seconds to ensure it's well mixed.
4. Serve the coconut water immediately or refrigerate for later use.

Nutritional Information (per serving):

- Carbs: 9g
- Sodium: 45mg
- Potassium: 600mg
- Phosphorus: 50mg
- Protein: 2g

Iced Coffee

Prep Time: 5 minutes | **Cook Time:** 5 minutes | **Servings:** 2

Ingredients:

- 2 cups brewed coffee, cooled
- 1 cup unsweetened almond milk
- 1 tablespoon granulated sweetener of choice (optional)
- Ice cubes

Instructions:

1. Brew 2 cups of coffee and allow it to cool to room temperature.
2. In a pitcher, put in the cooled brewed coffee with 1 cup of unsweetened almond milk.
3. If desired, add 1 tablespoon of your preferred granulated sweetener and stir until dissolved.
4. Fill two glasses with ice cubes.
5. Pour the coffee mixture over the ice cubes in each glass.
6. Stir adequately and serve immediately.

Nutritional Information (per serving):

- Carbs: 2g
- Sodium: 40mg
- Potassium: 80mg
- Phosphorus: 40mg
- Protein: 1g

Golden Milk

Prep Time: 5 minutes | **Cook Time:** 10 minutes | **Servings:** 2

Ingredients:

- 2 cups unsweetened almond milk
- 1 teaspoon ground turmeric
- 1/2 teaspoon ground cinnamon
- 1/4 teaspoon ground ginger
- 1 tablespoon honey (optional)
- Pinch of black pepper

Instructions:

1. In a small saucepan, combine 2 cups of unsweetened almond milk with 1 teaspoon of ground turmeric, 1/2 teaspoon of ground cinnamon, and 1/4 teaspoon of ground ginger.
2. Add a pinch of black pepper to the mixture. The black pepper helps with the absorption of turmeric.
3. Heat the mixture over medium-low heat, stirring frequently, for about 5-7 minutes until it's heated through but not boiling.
4. Take out the saucepan from the heat and stir in 1 tablespoon of honey, if desired, until dissolved.
5. Pour the golden milk into mugs and serve warm.

Nutritional Information (per serving):

- Carbs: 8g
- Sodium: 90mg
- Potassium: 150mg
- Phosphorus: 60mg
- Protein: 1g

Sparkling Water

Prep Time: 5 minutes | **Cook Time:** 0 minutes | **Servings:** 2

Ingredients:

- 2 cups cold water
- 1/2 cup sparkling water
- 1/2 lemon, sliced
- 1/2 lime, sliced
- Ice cubes

Instructions:

1. In a pitcher, combine 2 cups of cold water with 1/2 cup of sparkling water.
2. Add sliced 1/2 lemon and 1/2 lime to the pitcher.
3. Stir gently to mix the ingredients.
4. Fill two glasses with ice cubes.
5. Pour the sparkling water mixture into the glasses.
6. Garnish with additional lemon or lime slices if desired.
7. Serve immediately.

Nutritional Information (per serving):

- Carbs: 2g
- Sodium: 8mg
- Potassium: 45mg
- Phosphorus: 0mg
- Protein: 0g

Chai Latte

Prep Time: 5 minutes | **Cook Time:** 15 minutes | **Servings:** 2

Ingredients:

- 2 cups unsweetened almond milk
- 2 cinnamon sticks
- 4 whole cloves
- 4 cardamom pods, lightly crushed
- 1-inch piece of fresh ginger, sliced
- 2 black tea bags
- 1 tablespoon honey (optional)
- Ground cinnamon, for garnish (optional)

Instructions:

1. In a saucepan, combine 2 cups of unsweetened almond milk with 2 cinnamon sticks, 4 whole cloves, 4 lightly crushed cardamom pods, and sliced 1-inch piece of fresh ginger.
2. Bring the mixture to a simmer over medium heat, then reduce the heat to low and let it simmer gently for about 10 minutes to infuse the flavors.
3. Take out the saucepan from the heat and add 2 black tea bags. Steep for 3-5 minutes.
4. Take out the tea bags and strain the chai mixture through a fine mesh sieve to take out the spices.
5. Stir in 1 tablespoon of honey, if desired, until dissolved.
6. Pour the chai latte into mugs and sprinkle with ground cinnamon for garnish, if desired.
7. Serve hot.

Nutritional Information (per serving):

- Carbs: 8g
- Sodium: 90mg
- Potassium: 100mg
- Phosphorus: 60mg
- Protein: 1g

Hot Chocolate

Prep Time: 5 minutes | **Cook Time:** 10 minutes | **Servings:** 2

Ingredients:

- 2 cups unsweetened almond milk
- 2 tablespoons unsweetened cocoa powder
- 2 tablespoons granulated sweetener of choice (optional)
- 1/2 teaspoon vanilla extract
- Pinch of salt

Instructions:

1. In a small saucepan, combine 2 cups of unsweetened almond milk, 2 tablespoons of unsweetened cocoa powder, and 2 tablespoons of granulated sweetener of choice (if using).
2. Whisk the mixture over medium heat until the cocoa powder is fully dissolved and the milk is heated through, about 5-7 minutes.
3. Stir in 1/2 teaspoon of vanilla extract and a pinch of salt.
4. Continue to heat for an additional 2-3 minutes, stirring occasionally, until the hot chocolate is steaming hot but not boiling.
5. Take out the saucepan from the heat and pour the hot chocolate into mugs.
6. Serve immediately.

Nutritional Information (per serving):

- Carbs: 7g
- Sodium: 90mg
- Potassium: 150mg
- Phosphorus: 60mg
- Protein: 2g

Fresh Squeezed Juice

Prep Time: 10 minutes | **Cook Time:** 0 minutes | **Servings:** 2

Ingredients:

- 2 oranges
- 2 apples
- 1/2 lemon
- 1-inch piece of ginger

Instructions:

1. Wash all the fruits thoroughly under running water.
2. Cut the oranges and apples into quarters, removing any seeds.
3. Cut the half lemon into slices.
4. Peel the ginger and slice it into thin pieces.
5. In a juicer, juice the oranges, apples, lemon slices, and ginger.
6. Once all the fruits are juiced, stir the juice gently to put in the flavors.
7. Pour the fresh squeezed juice into glasses and serve immediately.

Nutritional Information (per serving):

- Carbs: 25g
- Sodium: 0mg
- Potassium: 270mg
- Phosphorus: 40mg
- Protein: 1g

Matcha Latte

Prep Time: 5 minutes | **Cook Time:** 5 minutes | **Servings:** 1

Ingredients:

- 1 teaspoon matcha powder
- 1 cup unsweetened almond milk
- 1 tablespoon honey (optional)
- 1/2 teaspoon vanilla extract

Instructions:

1. In a small saucepan, heat 1 cup of unsweetened almond milk over medium heat until warmed but not boiling.
2. In a bowl, whisk together 1 teaspoon of matcha powder with a small amount of hot water to form a smooth paste.
3. Pour the matcha paste into the warmed almond milk and whisk until well combined.
4. Stir in 1 tablespoon of honey (if using) and 1/2 teaspoon of vanilla extract.
5. Continue to heat the matcha latte mixture for an additional 1-2 minutes, stirring occasionally, until it reaches your desired temperature.
6. Pour the matcha latte into a mug and serve hot.

Nutritional Information (per serving):

- Carbs: 13g
- Sodium: 90mg
- Potassium: 180mg
- Phosphorus: 50mg
- Protein: 2g

Kombucha

Prep Time: 10 minutes | **Cook Time:** 10 minutes | Fermentation Time: 7-14 days | **Servings:** Variable

Ingredients:

- 1 SCOBY (symbiotic culture of bacteria and yeast)
- 1 cup white sugar
- 4 black tea bags
- 4 cups filtered water
- 1 cup starter tea (previously brewed kombucha)

Instructions:

1. Boil 4 cups of filtered water in a large pot. Once boiling, remove from heat and add 4 black tea bags. Let steep for 5-7 minutes.
2. Take out the tea bags and stir in 1 cup of white sugar until dissolved. Allow the sweetened tea to cool to room temperature.
3. Pour the cooled tea into a clean glass jar, leaving some space at the top. Add 1 cup of starter tea and gently place the SCOBY on top.
4. Cover the jar with a clean cloth or paper towel and secure it with a rubber band. Place the jar in a warm, dark place for 7-14 days to ferment.
5. After 7 days, taste the kombucha. If it's too sweet, let it ferment for a few more days. If it's too sour, it's ready to be bottled.
6. Carefully take out the SCOBY and set it aside. Pour the kombucha into glass bottles, leaving about an inch of space at the top.
7. Seal the bottles tightly and refrigerate to halt the fermentation process.
8. Serve the chilled kombucha and store any unused portion in the refrigerator.

Nutritional Information (per 8 oz serving):

- Carbs: 7g
- Sodium: 10mg
- Potassium: 20mg
- Phosphorus: 10mg
- Protein: 0g

Electrolyte Drink

Prep Time: 5 minutes | **Cook Time:** 0 minutes | **Servings:** 1

Ingredients:

- 1 cup coconut water
- 1/4 cup freshly squeezed orange juice
- 1/4 teaspoon sea salt
- 1 teaspoon honey or maple syrup (optional)
- Ice cubes

Instructions:

1. In a glass, combine 1 cup of coconut water with 1/4 cup of freshly squeezed orange juice.
2. Add 1/4 teaspoon of sea salt to the mixture and stir until dissolved.
3. Optionally, sweeten the electrolyte drink with 1 teaspoon of honey or maple syrup, stirring until fully incorporated.
4. Add ice cubes to the glass to chill the drink.
5. Stir adequately and serve immediately.

Nutritional Information (per serving):

- Carbs: 14g
- Sodium: 200mg
- Potassium: 470mg
- Phosphorus: 30mg
- Protein: 1g

Horchata

Prep Time: 10 minutes | **Cook Time:** 0 minutes | **Servings:** 4

Ingredients:

- 1 cup long-grain white rice
- 4 cups water
- 1 cinnamon stick
- 1/4 cup granulated sugar
- 1/2 teaspoon vanilla extract
- Ground cinnamon, for garnish (optional)

Instructions:

1. Rinse 1 cup of long-grain white rice under cold water until the water runs clear.
2. In a blender, put in the rinsed rice with 4 cups of water and 1 cinnamon stick. Blend until the rice is broken down but not completely smooth.
3. Let the rice mixture sit at room temperature for at least 30 minutes, or up to 2 hours, to allow the flavors to develop.
4. Strain the rice mixture through a fine mesh sieve or cheesecloth into a pitcher to take out the solids. Press down on the solids to extract as much liquid as possible.
5. Stir in 1/4 cup of granulated sugar and 1/2 teaspoon of vanilla extract until dissolved.
6. Chill the horchata in the refrigerator for at least 1 hour before serving.
7. Serve the horchata over ice cubes and garnish with ground cinnamon, if desired.

Nutritional Information (per serving):

- Carbs: 30g
- Sodium: 5mg
- Potassium: 40mg
- Phosphorus: 20mg
- Protein: 1g

Soy Milk

Prep Time: 10 minutes | **Cook Time:** 10 minutes | **Servings:** 4

Ingredients:

- 1 cup dried soybeans
- 4 cups water
- Sweetener of choice (optional), such as stevia or erythritol

Instructions:

1. Rinse 1 cup of dried soybeans under cold water and remove any debris.
2. Soak the soybeans in water overnight or for at least 8 hours.
3. After soaking, drain and rinse the soybeans thoroughly.
4. In a blender, put in the soaked soybeans with 4 cups of water.
5. Blend on high speed for 2-3 minutes until the mixture is smooth.
6. Strain the blended mixture through a nut milk bag or cheesecloth into a large bowl or pitcher, squeezing to extract as much liquid as possible.
7. Transfer the strained soy milk back into the blender and blend for an additional 1-2 minutes.
8. Optionally, sweeten the soy milk with your preferred sweetener, such as stevia or erythritol, and blend again until well combined.
9. Pour the soy milk into a clean container and refrigerate. It will keep for about 3-4 days.

Nutritional Information (per serving):

- Carbs: 4g
- Sodium: 10mg
- Potassium: 150mg
- Phosphorus: 70mg
- Protein: 7g

Conclusion

Congratulations on making it through the **30-Minute Renal Diet Cookbook**! We hope you have found a variety of delicious and easy-to-prepare meals that support your kidney health. As you continue your journey, here are some final tips for maintaining a renal-friendly diet and practical meal planning and preparation ideas to keep you on track.

Tips for Maintaining a Renal-Friendly Diet

Maintaining a renal-friendly diet involves consistent effort and mindful choices. Here are some practical tips to help you stay committed to your dietary goals:

1. **Stay Informed**: Keep up-to-date with the latest information about kidney health and dietary recommendations. Regularly consult your healthcare provider or a registered dietitian to ensure your diet meets your specific needs.

2. **Read Labels**: Always read food labels to check for sodium, potassium, and phosphorus content. Opt for products labeled "low-sodium," "no added salt," or "renal-friendly."

3. **Monitor Portions**: Pay attention to portion sizes, especially for foods high in potassium and phosphorus. Even healthy foods can become problematic if consumed in large quantities.

4. **Hydrate Wisely**: Drink adequate fluids as advised by your healthcare provider. Avoid sugary drinks, sodas, and high-potassium beverages like orange juice.

5. **Limit Processed Foods**: Processed and packaged foods often contain high levels of sodium and phosphorus additives. Choose fresh, whole foods whenever possible.

6. **Incorporate Variety**: Include a wide range of fruits, vegetables, proteins, and grains in your diet to ensure you get a balanced mix of nutrients without overloading on any one element.

7. **Stay Motivated**: Keep a food journal, set achievable goals, and celebrate your successes. Staying motivated will help you adhere to your diet and make positive lifestyle changes.

Meal Planning and Prep Ideas

Effective meal planning and preparation can make following a renal diet easier and more enjoyable. Here are some ideas to help you plan and prep your meals efficiently:

1. **Weekly Meal Plans**: Set aside time each week to plan your meals. Create a menu that includes breakfast, snacks, lunches, dinners, and even desserts. This will help you stay organized and avoid last-minute unhealthy choices.

2. **Create a Shopping List**: Based on your meal plan, make a detailed shopping list. Stick to the list and ensure you have all the ingredients needed for the week to avoid buying unnecessary items.

3. **Prep Ahead**: Dedicate a few hours each week to prepping ingredients. Wash and chop vegetables, cook grains, and portion out proteins. Store these prepped items in clear containers for easy access.

4. **Batch Cooking**: Cook larger portions of your favorite renal-friendly meals and freeze individual servings. This is a great way to ensure you always have a quick, healthy meal ready on busy days.

5. **Use Versatile Ingredients**: Choose ingredients that can be used in multiple dishes. For instance, you can use roasted chicken in salads, wraps, and main dishes, saving time and reducing food waste.

6. **Organize Your Kitchen**: Keep your kitchen well-organized with labeled containers, clear storage solutions, and a designated space for renal-friendly staples. An organized kitchen makes cooking more efficient and enjoyable.

7. **Experiment and Adapt**: Don't be afraid to try new recipes and adapt them to your dietary needs. The more you experiment, the more confident you'll become in creating delicious and compliant meals.

By integrating these tips and ideas into your routine, you can maintain a renal-friendly diet without sacrificing flavor or variety. Remember, the key to success is planning, preparation, and a positive attitude.

Finally, thank you for choosing the *30-Minute Renal Diet Cookbook*. We hope it becomes a valuable resource in your kitchen, helping you enjoy quick, healthy, and kidney-friendly meals every day. Here's to your health and happiness!

Recipes Index

A

Almond Milk 99

Angel Food Cake 81

Apple Cinnamon Bars 89

Apple Cinnamon Oatmeal 10

Apple Slices with Peanut Butter 60

Avocado Toast 16

B

Baked Chicken Parmesan 53

Baked Cod 48

Baked Salmon 41

Banana Ice Cream 82

Banana Nut Muffins 12

Beef and Barley Soup 39

Beef and Broccoli 55

Beef Stew 47

Berry Crisp 78

Berry Smoothie Bowl 91

Black Bean Soup 29

Blueberry Pancakes 11

Breakfast Casserole 20

Breakfast Quesadilla 17

C

Caprese Salad 31

Carrot Sticks with Hummus 66

Chai Latte 106

Cheese and Crackers 63

Chia Seed Pudding 94

Chicken and Rice Soup 36

Chicken Caesar Salad 24

Chicken Noodle Soup 30

Chicken Stir-Fry 46

Chocolate Avocado Mousse 84

Chocolate Covered Strawberries 93

Cinnamon Raisin French Toast 9

Coconut Macaroons 90

Coconut Water 102

Cottage Cheese 67

E

Edamame 71

Egg Salad Sandwich 32

Electrolyte Drink 111

F

Fresh Squeezed Juice 108

Fruit Infused Water 98

Fruit Salad 70

G

Golden Milk 104

Greek Chickpea Salad 34

Greek Salad 23

Greek Yogurt 62

Greek Yogurt Cheesecake 92

Greek Yogurt Parfait 13

Green Smoothie 96

Grilled Shrimp Skewers 44

H

Horchata 112

Hot Chocolate 107

I

Iced Coffee 103

Iced Herbal Tea 97

K

Kombucha 110

L

Lemon Garlic Tilapia 54

Lemon Herb Chicken 42

Lemon Poppy Seed Muffins 85

Lentil Curry 58

Lentil Soup 27

M

Matcha Latte 109

Minestrone Soup 28

Mixed Nuts 65

Mushroom Risotto 56

O

Oatmeal Raisin Cookies 87

P

Peach Cobbler 88

Peanut Butter Banana Bites 75

Poached Pears 79

Popcorn 68

Pork Tenderloin 49

Pretzels 72

Protein Shake 100

Pumpkin Pie 86

Q

Quinoa Salad 25

R

Ratatouille 45

Rice Cakes with Hummus 64

Rice Pudding 80

Roasted Chickpeas 73

Roasted Vegetable Wrap 38

S

Sliced Cucumber with Lemon 69

Soy Milk 113

Sparkling Water 105

Spinach and Feta Stuffed Chicken 57

Spinach and Lentil Salad 37

Spinach and Mushroom Omelette 18

Strawberry Banana Smoothie 15

Strawberry Sorbet 83

Stuffed Peppers 51

T

Tomato Basil Soup 33

Trail Mix 61

Tuna Salad 26

Turkey and Avocado Wrap 22

Turkey Chili 43

Turkey Meatballs 52

V

Vegetable Barley Soup 35

Vegetable Frittata 14

Vegetable Juice 101

Vegetable Stir-Fry 50

Veggie Chips 76

W

Whole Grain Waffles 19

Y

Yogurt and Berry Bowl 8

Yogurt Bark 74

www.ingramcontent.com/pod-product-compliance
Lightning Source LLC
Chambersburg PA
CBHW082208220526
45470CB00010B/3092